HOW TO SLEEP BETTER

The detailed notes pertaining to this book are available on the HarperCollins *Publishers* India website. Scan this QR code to access the same.

HOW TO SLEEP BETTER

The Miraculous Ten-step
Protocol to Recharge
Your Mind and Body

DEEPA KANNAN

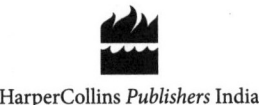

HarperCollins *Publishers* India

First published in India by HarperCollins *Publishers* 2023
4th Floor, Tower A, Building No. 10, DLF Cyber City,
DLF Phase II, Gurugram, Haryana – 122002
www.harpercollins.co.in

2 4 6 8 10 9 7 5 3 1

Copyright © Deepa Kannan 2023

P-ISBN: 978-93-5699-563-5
E-ISBN: 978-93-5699-564-2

The views and opinions expressed in this book are the author's own
and the facts are as reported by her, and the publishers are not in
any way liable for the same.

Deepa Kannan asserts the moral right
to be identified as the author of this work.

All rights reserved. No part of this publication may be reproduced,
stored in a retrieval system, or transmitted, in any form or by any means,
electronic, mechanical, photocopying, recording or otherwise,
without the prior permission of the publishers.

Typeset in 11/14.5 Bembo Std at
Manipal Technologies Limited, Manipal

Printed and bound at
Thomson Press (India) Ltd

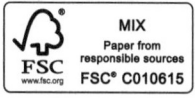

This book is produced from independently certified FSC® paper
to ensure responsible forest management.

To Shyam, my guiding light and soul connection
To Omkar, my ultimate divine purpose
and
In fond memory of Appa

Disclaimer

This book, unless otherwise noted, is based upon the opinions, ideas and experiences of the author, who is an allied functional medicine practitioner and Ayurvedic health counsellor. Names, characters, events and incidents in this book have been changed to protect identities. Any resemblance to actual persons, living or dead, or actual events is purely coincidental. It is intended to provide helpful and informative material on the subject matter covered. The author is not acting in the capacity of a doctor or a registered physician/dietitian, and is not rendering any professional, healthcare or medical services through this book. The information in this book is not intended as a substitute for medical advice and counselling, or as treatment/cure for any particular health condition. The advice and tools contained herein may not be suitable for your situation. Any medical questions regarding contraindications and precautions or any questions on whether or not the reader is to proceed with any practices provided in this book should be referred to qualified health professionals before adopting the same. The author specifically disclaims any responsibility for any liability, loss or risk, personal or otherwise, which may be incurred as a direct or indirect consequence of the use of this book or the application/adoption of any of the information provided in this book.

Contents

Foreword by Mark Hyman	xi
Foreword by Nanditha Krishna	xiii
Introduction	xv

Part 1
Understanding Sleep

1.	How and Why We Sleep	1
2.	Indriyas: Your Instruments of True Knowledge	6

Part 2
The First Sense: Sight

3.	Sight, Light and Vision	10
4.	The Circadian Rhythm	17
5.	Your Inner Clock	24
6.	Therapies for Your Sense of Sight	28

Part 3
The Second Sense: Sound

7.	Sound, Vata Dosha and Adrenals	38

8. Adrenal Function, the HPA Axis and Sound — 45
9. Therapies for Your Sense of Sound — 52

Part 4
The Third Sense: Smell

10. Smell, Emotions and Memories — 58
11. Breath: The Symbol of Prana — 64
12. The Glymphatic System and Sleep — 67
13. Therapies for Your Sense of Smell — 76

Part 5
The Fourth Sense: Touch

14. Touch, Connection and Oxytocin — 83
15. The Seesaw of Oxytocin and Cortisol — 89
16. Therapies for Your Sense of Touch — 96

Part 6
The Fifth Sense: Taste

17. Taste, Gratitude and Fasting — 102
18. The Vagus Nerve, Fasting and Sleep — 108
19. The Six Tastes — 114
20. Therapies for Your Sense of Taste — 120

Part 7
The Sixth Sense: Detoxification

21. Digestion and Detoxification — 124
22. Agni for Great Sleep — 134

Contents

23. The Liver and Detoxification	137
24. Therapies for Your Sense of Detoxification	146

Part 8
The Seventh Sense: Uro Reproduction

25. The Urinary System and Vata Dosha	153
26. How Hormones Impact Sleep	161
27. Sexual Energy and Vitality	170
28. Therapies for Your Sense of Uro-Reproduction	172

Part 9
The Eight Sense: Locomotion

29. Locomotion, Movement and the Circadian Rhythm	176
30. Movement for Great Sleep	184
31. Therapies for Your Sense of Locomotion	191

Part 10
The Ninth Sense: Grasping

32. Grasping, Strength and Nerves	195
33. Hands, Muscles and Nerves	200
34. Pain and Sleep	204
35. Therapies for Your Sense of Grasping	209

Part 11
The Tenth Sense: Speech

36. Speech, the Thyroid Gland and Resilience	213
37. The Miracle Gland: The Thyroid	219
38. Therapies for Your Sense of Speech	228

Part 12
The Ten-sense Protocol

Week 1	238
Week 2	250
Week 3	262
Week 4	268
39. How to Choose a Sleeping Position	278
40. Eating for Good Sleep	282
Resources	287
Acknowledgments	289
Notes	295

Foreword

Mark Hyman

Quality sleep is one of the most important pillars of health, but is often ignored. According to recent studies, one out of every three adults in the US reports getting less than the recommended amount of sleep necessary for optimal health. Sleep hygiene is as important to overall health as diet—and possibly more so. Over time, poor sleep can negatively impact every other facet of health, including cognition, energy, hormones, mood and even our ability to heal from chronic inflammation.

If you are one of the many millions of people who have trouble getting a good night's sleep or feel tired all the time—and are stressed out because you've tried everything—don't lose hope.

The truth is, sleep exists on a continuum. On one side are those who have a diagnosed sleeping disorder; on the other side are those who sleep like a baby every single night. Most of us fall somewhere in between these two extremes, and when sleep troubles crop up, we're left with no other option than trying various medications and internet cure-alls with the fleeting hope that one of them might work. This is truly an injustice because these are far from the only, or even the best, solutions available—if you know where to look.

This is where functional medicine and Ayurveda come in. Functional medicine uses the latest scientific understanding about how our genetics, environment and lifestyle interact together to diagnose, treat diseases based on patterns of imbalance and dysfunction. Ayurveda looks at the individual through specific patterns in the combination of three energies. Both take into account the web-like relationships between all aspects of a person's health and offer plenty of solutions that bring the power back into your hands.

That is why I am so excited to introduce you to this groundbreaking new book on sleep. This book combines ancient practices with the science of Functional Medicine to help you unlock the secrets of restful, rejuvenating sleep. It offers practical tips, tools and techniques you can use to optimize your sleep, and wake up feeling refreshed, energized and ready to tackle the day ahead.

In this book, you'll gain insight into Deepa's intuitive understanding of the interconnectedness of the body, learn from her how to address the wide range of root causes of sleep challenges and access tools you can utilize from the comfort of your own home. She lays out the key pieces of information you'll need to move from chronic sleep challenges to truly deep and healing sleep.

So, whether you're dealing with chronic insomnia or simply looking to improve your overall sleep quality, this book is an invaluable resource that can help you achieve the deep, restorative sleep that your body and mind deserve. I'm proud of you for taking the first step toward moving from helplessness to empowerment by trusting your instincts and picking up this book.

Foreword

Nanditha Krishna

'What hath night to do with sleep?' asked John Milton. Everything.

When we shut our eyes to go to sleep, we create the same environment as the night, a period of darkness, silence and peace.

Achieving peace through deep sleep is the goal of every person, but achieving sleep is itself difficult for many. Deepa is an allied functional medicinal practitioner and Ayurvedic health counsellor who tries to help the reader 'sleep better'. Issues like sleep deprivation, depression and lifestyle affect our internal clock, the 'circadian rhythm' that plays a vital role in all body systems and functions, and regulates our wakefulness and sleep rhythms which, in turn, respond to changing light and sound. India's legends include people who were blessed with or without sleep. The most famous was Kumbakarna, who slept for six months at a time and woke up for just one day to eat his fill before going back to sleep. Lakshmana was given the divine boon by the goddess of sleep, Nidra, whereby he stayed awake for fourteen years to protect Rama, while his wife Urmila slept on his behalf and her own. In nature, butterflies don't sleep, they merely rest with their eyes open. A walrus can stay awake for 84 hours, while tilapia fish can stay without sleep for 22 weeks after birth. Nature has created animals for the day and for the night. This way, the pressure by predators was limited. Nocturnal creatures are active at night. Crepuscular creatures are active at dawn and dusk. Diurnal beings, including humans, are active during the day, and in sync with the earth's diurnal rhythm of light and darkness.

Deepa has chosen to share her knowledge, acquired over the years. I congratulate her for taking on an essential but neglected part of our lives, especially in these days of television and mobile phones which have taken over our waking and sleeping hours. Finally, to quote Charaka (21/36), 'Happiness, misery, nourishment, emaciation, strength, weakness, virility, sterility, knowledge, ignorance, life and death—all these occur depending on proper or improper sleep.'

Introduction

My childhood was full of bedtime stories and fairy tales, some of which were about sleeping. From Hindu mythology came Kumbakarna, Ravana's brother in the Ramayana, who was known for his superhuman strength and his tendency to sleep for months at a stretch. Greek mythology has Hypnos, god of sleep, from whose name the word 'hypnosis' is derived. In fairy tales, we have Sleeping Beauty, who was in a deep slumber until her prince arrived.

Yet, when it came to my own life, I was never told to prioritize sleep. I'll come to my story later, but what I want you to know is that my health issues were persistent and debilitating. I suffered a great deal, but I also had to go through life every day, simply because I could not afford to not do so.

You might be struggling with some impact on your mind and body from poor sleep. Do you feel pressured to perform efficiently even after a night of poor sleep? Do you have digestive distress that makes you severely uncomfortable through the day? Do you succumb to frequent infections and challenges to your immune system? Is your overall health getting destroyed, day by day? Are you struggling to cope emotionally and mentally? Is perpetual anxiety spinning your mind into a whirlwind of panic and confusion?

What if I told you that there is a framework available that will allow you to explore almost every possible root cause of poor sleep, and that it is based on a wonderful synergy between the cutting-edge science of functional medicine and the ancient Eastern wisdom of yoga and Ayurveda?

Is This Book for You?

Everything in this book is based on a deeper understanding of what is present within you. Think of this book as a unique system which will allow you to be the best version of yourself. You will be able to transform the state of your sleep, as well as your whole life.

This is the right book for you if you find yourself resonating with any of these statements:

1. You feel like you have so much to achieve, but you simply do not have the energy to do much.
2. You struggle with severe digestive challenges that drain you of whatever energy you have.
3. You want to be more alert, focused, creative and driven, but a sudden night of terrible sleep occurs just before a major event and destroys that focus.
4. You have tried every possible sleep gimmick out there and nothing works for you personally.
5. You have started to believe that poor sleep is a part of who you are and that it will never ever change for the better.

6. You are constantly challenged by infections of every kind that spiral you into a loop of medication, digestive destruction and deep anxiety.
7. You want to be happy while spending time with your family, but the continuous lack of sleep is making you frequently weepy or angry.
8. You have an excessive appetite and eat a lot of the wrong kinds of food because your body is forever trying to compensate for the lack of energy from poor sleep.
9. You struggle with hormonal imbalance that makes you suffer from acne, mood swings and weight gain.
10. You are battling against numbing anxiety and even deeper depression because your brain feels tired.
11. You are struggling with symptoms of early menopause that is affecting your mood, libido and energy. Yet, physiologically, you should not be in this phase for a few more years.
12. You are not physically or emotionally enjoying your relationship with your partner and this is hurting you deeply.
13. You feel constant fatigue, but nothing seems to change that.
14. You think that you are meant to suffer this way forever because you can see no other way beyond this.

This book is for almost everyone at some point in time in their lives. The truth is, irrespective of practically everything else, if you struggle with sleep, perpetually or sporadically, this book is going to provide you with frameworks and tools that will empower you. It is also entirely up to you how you approach or use this information. While there will be protocols for you, feel free to adapt them to suit your needs. Once you have read the whole book, you will gain a deeper understanding of your ten senses, as well as visionary plans and protocols for sleep, and that spark of inspiration will transform your sleep and your life. This book will also serve you if you are a healthcare practitioner. If you have clients that struggle with sleep, this can truly be a guidebook for them as well.

This book:

1. Will clear all confusion about sleep, and teach you how sleep affects every system and organ in your body, so that you will have the tools to positively impact your whole body through better sleep.
2. Will give you a blueprint to restore sleep to create a better life with a greater vision for yourself.
3. Will provide you with the tools you need to have better relationships and greater pleasure.
4. Will teach you to take charge of your sleep and your life.
5. Will give you the knowledge that you require and the freedom to use that knowledge in ways that are personal, meaningful, applicable and useful to you specifically, or to your clients if you are a healthcare practitioner.

In every chapter, you will learn specific information. You might find yourself resonating with one chapter more than another, and this will also reveal specific vulnerabilities in yourself. Think of this discovery as deeply enlightening, for it will also show you the path ahead specifically for you. By writing this book, I have attempted to solve your problems with sleep—whatever they are!

I explore sleep in the deepest manner, looking at root causes before providing solutions. Its greatest quality is its depth and the compelling characters whose stories you will learn through case studies. By sharing stories, all the principles of each section are explored through their impact on people's lives. This will allow you to experience a eureka moment where you will feel understood and validated, leaving you with a sense of hope. A sleep whisperer is someone who has the capacity of taming anyone—even a person with the most unmanageable sleep. I believe this book will be a sleep whisperer to you, empowering you with the knowledge you need to transform your sleep and your life.

While it is wonderful that there is rising awareness and growth of this industry, along with better tools to support sleep recovery, I think it is very important to also navigate sleep's relationship with food and nutrients, as well as to explore tools and therapies that we can use safely. For many who lie within the gap between having a diagnosed sleep disorder and great sleep, these can be transformational. They can also be supportive strategies alongside other interventions, if they are required.

My Story

I'm in my late forties and, after four decades of suffering from some of the worst health crises, I can confidently say that sleep is a great tool to support overall health. I can either think that I wished I had had the knowledge I have today back then or I can look back in some gratitude at all that I faced, as most of my struggles led me to the path on which I am today.

I got married in my early twenties, was divorced by the time I was thirty and remarried a yogi. My son was born with a rare adrenal disorder called salt-wasting Congenital Adrenal Hyperplasia, from which he almost died at three weeks. Children born with this condition do not produce cortisol and aldosterone. They can die under multiple situations through dehydration. He had seizures, multiple dehydration episodes and hospital visits, and was highly susceptible to many viral infections due to him being steroid-dependent. My understanding of the adrenal system due to my son's condition is what gave me the depth of understanding required to write a book on sleep. While trauma and fear can keep you from sleeping, if you are a mother, you know how your sleep becomes the last priority. Life is a perpetual journey, never a destination.

Speaking about the gap in the sleep-resolution matrix has been on my mind for a while now. There is something missing in the sleep-care paradigm. The chasm that exists between someone who can be diagnosed with a chronic sleep disorder and someone who has great sleep is wide. Millions exist in this gap. There is so much we can do to improve our sleep if we fall into this gap or even if we do have a sleep condition, provided we work alongside the medical model. We cannot deny that interventions like diet and ancient therapies work to help us. Can we put them aside because there isn't enough research on them? That would be an injustice to ourselves now, wouldn't it?

You'll notice that I have linked several research articles and studies in each chapter, but I do want to say something about research versus the individual. Coming from a long-standing yoga background, I realized that not everything needs to be validated by research. There is a world of difference between research on yoga and meditation now and twenty-five years ago, when I started teaching.

I ask you to look at research while also embracing the possibility that there can be wisdom in ancient texts. My focus has been on serving you in the best way possible. At times, research can also be contradictory, confusing and even discouraging. It can get so complex that you could feel lost if you are not able to understand its subtleties and intricacies. What I set out to do was to make things as simple as possible with tools that you can use for yourself. We have been trained to analyse separate components in isolation, never the overall effect on ourselves based on our individual body constitution, season, location or present state of health. I did not want to miss this big picture, so I only attempted to correlate some of my intuitive and experiential knowledge with interesting data out there. You can do so much to make a difference by just trying something and being mindful of your body's response.

PART 1

Understanding Sleep

1

How and Why We Sleep

Fourteen years ago, I thought I was starting a new phase of life when I gave birth to my little boy. He was three weeks old when I ran into the emergency room not knowing what was happening, handing over a baby who had shrivelled up overnight and turned dark before my eyes. I watched in horror as they wheeled him away as fear clutched at my heart. A few hours later, I asked the senior doctor if my baby was going to die. I learned that he had an adrenal disorder for life.

During that first year, the thought that sleep was important for my well-being never even crossed my mind. In the frequent trips to the emergency room, I felt my health slipping away. I noticed my immune system weaken as infections became more frequent. There began several years of chronic ill health. It took me five more years to understand how our body heals in sleep, and how pivotal sleep is to health of the body and mind.

Stages of Sleep

Your brain releases neurotransmitters, or nerve-signalling hormones, which decide if you are awake or asleep. Your brain does not sleep. When you are asleep, some parts of your brain are very much awake, guiding vital actions. When it comes to the connection between sleep and the upkeep of different parts of your body, you will see that you simply cannot get away with continuous lack of quality sleep. Sleep has many stages, and knowing the different stages is important to understanding why you need continuous and uninterrupted sleep.

During a good night's sleep, you pass through different stages of sleep, known as 1, 2, 3, 4 and Rapid Eye Movement (REM). You move from 1 towards REM, and then the cycle repeats. A majority of sleeping time is spent in stage 2.

The Stages of Sleep

1. **Non-REM Stage 1** sleep is extremely light. It occurs when you are drifting between waking and sleeping, and thus are still impacted by the feedback from your senses. You can also experience muscular movement or twitches. It is a phase where you start slowing down your heart rate and breathing in preparation for sleep.
2. **Non-REM Stage 2** sleep is a state where your eye movements reduce and even your brain activity slows down. Heart rate, breathing, eye movements and brain activity start slowing down. Non-REM stages 1 and 2 make up the bulk of your total sleep.
3. During **Non-REM Stage 3** of your sleep, your brain starts to produce slow waves, called delta waves, interspersed with some rapid ones. There is hardly any eye or muscle movement, and most people don't wake up easily from this stage of sleep. This phase is considered actual deep sleep.

4. In **Non-REM Stage 4**, mostly delta waves of deep sleep are produced. Once again, there is no eye or muscle movement and it is rare for someone to wake up easily from this state. Vital signs and brain waves are at the lowest. This is also the stage when young children are prone to bedwetting.
5. In **REM** sleep, breathing can become irregular, your eyes may twitch, your muscles may move involuntarily, your heart rate and blood pressure could rise and, when you wake up suddenly from REM sleep, you can recall bizarre dreams. This stage of sleep is also considered to be deep sleep, but the body's vital signs and brain waves are similar to those of waking up.

All deep sleep stages are critical for repair, brain healing, memory formation, hormone optimization and detoxification. It is not how much you sleep, but how much you stay in deep sleep that matters. Typically, stages 1 and 2 should be around 55 per cent, stages 3 and 4 around 20 per cent, and REM 25 per cent. This ratio means that you have entered all stages of sleep adequately to repair and rejuvenate. However, I would caution against getting caught up with sleep-tracking devices.

The Devastating Impact of Chronic Sleep Deprivation

I know so many people who just laugh off their poor sleep patterns. Is poor sleep not such a big deal? Can you get away with not getting deep and restorative sleep? Some of the functional impacts of poor sleep include the following:

1. Lack of sleep is a stressor, which can impact your digestion and make any pre-existing symptoms much worse. One night

of poor sleep also raises ghrelin, the hunger hormone, so you feel unnatural hunger, and lowers leptin, the satiety hormone, so that no amount of food will make you feel full. It's not your fault for craving foods rich in sugar or salt after a poor night's sleep.

2. It can slow down the movement of peristalsis within your intestine, leading to constipation, nutrient malabsorption, fermentation, yeast overgrowth and build-up of toxic waste.
3. It also reduces melatonin and low melatonin has been linked to permeability of our intestine.
4. Low melatonin reduces antioxidant activity in the brain, and can create oxidative stress and free radical damage, or, in simple words, it can make you age quickly.
5. Sleep deprivation prevents your liver from restoring itself, putting a strain on it, and resulting in a build-up of exogenous and endogenous toxins.
6. Lack of sleep reduces your white blood cells and suppresses your immunity. In fact, it can truly be said that lack of sleep is one of the biggest enemies of your immune system. This then makes you susceptible to attack from pathogens and more prone to infections.
7. Some of you may have many genes that are either inherited from your ancestors and make you prone to something, or you may have polymorphisms. While not all those genes express, lack of sleep is an epigenetic factor and can trigger gene expression.
8. Lack of sleep can negatively impact everything from insulin to cortisol, from thyroid to oestrogen, progesterone and testosterone, and from leptin to ghrelin.
9. Cerebral spinal fluid is a clear fluid protecting your brain within the cranium. In deep sleep, it washes toxins and

metabolic by-products from your brain via the glymphatic system. The brain can deteriorate when it does not undergo this regular cleaning.

> **Did you know ...**
>
> 1. 10–30 per cent of adults can struggle with chronic insomnia.[1]
> 2. Women can have up to 40 per cent higher risk for insomnia.[2]
> 3. Hormonal shifts and PMS impact sleep twice as much.[3]
> 4. 75 per cent of adults with depression also suffer from insomnia.[4]
> 5. Drinking alcohol disturbs sleep in both genders, depending on dosage.[5]
> 6. 80 per cent of people who take prescription sleep medication also report oversleeping, and experiencing a lack of focus and grogginess.[6]

2

Indriyas: Your Instruments of True Knowledge

If you have a connection to yoga or Ayurveda, or have been fascinated by Eastern traditions and ancient wisdom, you might be familiar with the ten senses. The ten senses of sleep came to me in a moment of intuition. It is built upon the idea of the ten indriyas. As you'll see as we go along, the ten senses are simply a foundation or a framework. Once you have a firm understanding of what they are, you'll start to understand how you can use them to regain your vitality, health and sleep. I advise you to read the book from start to finish the first time. After that, you can flip through to the section or sections that are most useful to you.

Five Senses Enter, Five Senses Exit

Imagine yourself as a house with ten doors, in which five allow what is outside to come in and the other five let what is inside go out. This is the simplest explanation of the ten indriyas.

The word 'indriyas' comes from Sanskrit and its literal translation means 'belonging to Indra'. Indra, the king of the gods, is frequently depicted as holding the vajra or the thunderbolt. Think about what this represents symbolically; think about how quickly your sense organs work, almost at the speed of lightning. The ten indriyas are divided into two categories: Jnana indriyas and karma indriyas.

Jnana indriyas are the five sense organs that you are already familiar with—that is, the eyes, nose, tongue, ears and skin, which allow you to see, smell, taste, hear and touch respectively. Think of them as sense organs to enter your body.

Then, the **karma indriyas** are exit organs, allowing you to move from your body and outside of yourself. These are the mouth, hands, feet, genitals and the rectum. They allow you to experience speech, dexterity, locomotion, reproduction and excretion. Karma indriyas are designed—or rather, they are designated—to perform certain actions. There are several texts that describe the indriyas. Below are two sources.

Sarada Tilaka, a text from the earlier times of the Tantric era, is written by Sri Lakshmana Desikendra, a saint-scholar who lived in Maharashtra, near present-day Nasik. His ancestors were scholars and tantra pandits. The book is an in-depth analysis and exploration of the origins of speech, the five elements, the five principles of the atom, etc. There is a verse that describes the ten senses in it: They are also described in the Ayurvedic text *Charaka Samhita*, among others.

Jnanendriyaani Srtotra Twak Drik Jihwa Nasika Viduhu
Jnanendriyaartha Shabdaadya Smritha Karmendriyanyapi
Vaak Paani Paada Paayuandu Samnyanya Hur Maneeshinaha
Vajanadanagadhayo Visargaananda Samyudaha

This means:

Ear, skin, eyes, mouth, and nose are the pancha indriyas through which you experience sound, touch, sight, taste and smell. Mouth, hands, leg, genitals, and rectum are the karma indriyas through which you experience speech, action, locomotion, procreation, and excretion. All these provide bliss.

In the Bhagavad Gita, chapter 13, verses 6–7, the indriyas are spoken about:

Maha-bhutany ahankaro
Buddhir avyaktam eva ca
Indriyani dasaikam ca
Pancha cendriya gocarah
Icha dvesam sukham duhkam
Sanghatas cetana dhrtih
Etat kshetram samasena
Sa vikaram udahrtam

The kshetram and its modifications are composed of the unmanifested Prakriti, the five cosmic elements, the ten senses, the one-sense mind, intelligence, ego and the five objects of the senses, which are desire, hate, pleasure, pain, aggregation, consciousness and persistence.

Is this new to you? Stay with me.

Remember that we might use the term 'ten senses' throughout the book. By using the term, we are talking about much more than just the anatomical perception of senses. We explore it from a space which is more comprehensive, where we derive its meanings from ancient traditions and apply it to modern science, bringing them together in a way you can easily understand.

The Ten-sense Promise

The ten-sense protocol is a model or a guideline that can reinvent the science of understanding sleep. It should be a catalyst to drive you towards reclaiming your sleep and your life. The protocol will help you navigate various vulnerable areas of poor sleep. Once you understand my blueprint, you will be able to make it work for you in your own unique way. When you uncover vulnerable senses, never allow them to frustrate you. The information here should feel enlightening and liberating.

Once you discover the frameworks and tools, you will positively wonder at some of the information, and feel that you should have known this many years ago! I will show you how you can build a plan that works synergistically between science and symbolism to offer you a chance to restore great sleep and ensure a better future. Now is the time for change. Act now.

PART 2

The First Sense: Sight

3

Sight, Light and Vision

Your eyes are your sense organ for sight. They bring you wonderful feedback from the outside world. They allow you to perceive and evaluate what you see, which can include form, colour, size and much more. The eyes connect you to your space, and they symbolize darkness and night.

Chronobiology is a field of science that examines periodic or cyclical phenomena in all living organisms. It studies how they adapt to solar and lunar rhythms that exist in nature, and their link to time. Imagine yourself to be another Alice in this fascinating chapter!

Sight and Poor Sleep Are Connected

Amara came to see me for various inflammatory challenges. She was in her early forties and had been diagnosed with optic neuritis, which is inflammation of the eyes that damages the optic nerve. Optic nerves are nerve fibres that help to transmit vital visual information from the eyes to the brain. Those who suffer from the condition experience pain, temporary loss of vision and what is called dry eyes, which occur when you do not produce enough tears. Tears help protect your eyes from irritants and infections.

Anyway, Amara had been struggling for many years. She had consulted many systems of medicine, but nothing had helped.

I asked her, 'How is your sleep?'

She replied, 'It's not too bad. I haven't had a full night's sleep in a long time, but I get by. The nights when it's very bad, I take some medication to help me sleep.'

She said that she slept just enough or not enough, slept for seven hours usually, had poor quality of sleep, was tired most days and sometimes remembered her dreams. She had blurred vision, dry eyes and eye strain.

She had a history of antibiotics consumption which was beyond the usual. This was my first clue about what was going on within her body. When there is such an aggressive use of antibiotics, then the chances of the gut being impacted are very high. When the gut is impacted, then the gut walls become permeable—a syndrome called leaky gut.

I asked her, 'Do you struggle to fall asleep? Or do you sleep, wake up and struggle to go back to sleep? What time do you go to bed?'

She replied, 'I go to bed by about midnight and fall asleep by around one in the morning.'

'Why do you go to bed so late?'

'That's not late!' she exclaimed.

Amara ate her dinner past 10 p.m. Then she flipped through channels and watched multiple television shows on Netflix, which were rather exciting. Once she started, she always struggled to stop. She went through a couple of episodes each night.

I asked her to show me a picture of her space. It was a dark room, with a few recliners. When she lay on one of them after dinner, she focused on the flashing lights from an exciting TV show. Then she lay tossing and turning in her bed, stressed by the fact she could not sleep and that she had to wake up in the morning to go to work. Eventually, she gave in to the medication and fell into an exhausted sleep, only to wake up in a trance.

Understanding Your Eyes and the Sense of Sight

I've had severe myopia since I was seven years old. So does my son. As I grew up, my vision became so bad that I could not see a few feet in front of me when I woke up. It was frustrating. Many years later, I had laser surgery done on my eyes and was left with great vision. However, when my problems with sleep started, I found that I was particularly sensitive to any source of light in a dark room—however small or dim it was. My husband even scolded me one day when I asked him to apply dark insulation tape to a glimmer of light and said I was acting like a sleep diva! I really have no idea if that surgery impacted anything in my eyes. Were my eyes now extra sensitive or was I that way all along? I do know that I am immensely sensitive to light. It's possible that some people are more sensitive than others. We can only speculate on the reasons behind this. Recently, when I asked my ophthalmologist about this, he felt it was highly possible.

There are so many reasons why your circadian rhythm might be more prone to disruption, beyond just the time you wake up and go to sleep. I know that most research in this area looks at factors such as wavelength, brightness of light and time, but I want to instead take you through the health of your eyes and situations where one person is affected more than another by it. Research shows fascinating connections between the health of the eyes and sleep.

The Environment of Your Eyes: Your Ocular Microbiome

Did you know that your eyes have their own microbiome? A microbiome is an inner ecosystem within your body, which exists in your gut, oral cavity, skin, organs, blood, mucosa and eyes, where microbes, virus and fungi live together, mostly in harmony.

Your microbiome controls how your body manages inflammation and how you maintain the integrity of the walls of the gut. It also controls brain chemistry, vital nutrient levels, hormones, metabolism, absorption, sleep and the circadian rhythm of your body.

In 2009, Valery Shestopalov, PhD, professor of biochemistry and cell biology at the Bascom Palmer Eye Institute at the University of Miami, discovered bacteria in healthy eyes. Until then, the belief was that the eyes did not hold microbial life due to tears and blinking washing them away, but his tests revealed that all the exposed mucosa was populated. It led him to begin the Ocular Microbiome Project,[7] which then revealed that people had a variety of bacteria in this ocular microbiome. When the cornea was infected, however, only a few bacteria existed, revealing the huge role of the ocular microbiome in the health of the eyes.

> **How Swimming in the Pool Affects Your Eyes**
>
> Unlike other microbiomes of the body, the composition of the ocular surface can be impacted by oxygen levels and pH, and can influence the bacterial community, which can then impact your eyes in various ways, including the occurrence of dry eyes. Could swimming in a pool with chlorine impact your ocular microbiome and make you more susceptible to inflammation in your eyes? It is possible. However, swimming is an amazing form of movement. Wear protective goggles the next time you swim and it will help preserve the integrity of your ocular microbiome.

What Role Do the Mucous Membranes Play?

Your immune system has many layers, but the first line of defence is your skin. Mucous membranes line parts of your body and coat some organs. They consist of a very thin layer of skin or epithelial cells and secrete mucous, which blocks pathogens from entering your body and prevents certain parts of your body from becoming dehydrated. Healthy mucosae play a big role in the health of your eyes.

You'll also understand later in this book how excess vata dosha can increase dryness in the whole body, including the eyes.

The Brain and Eye Connection

Within your brain, your cerebrum, or the forebrain, is considered the primary organ of your nervous system. The largest part of your brain, it occupies the whole upper part of your skull. The cerebrum is irregular and covered with grooves that serve to increase the brain's surface area. Some folds differ from brain to brain, but some are constant, of which one is the occipital lobe. Your occipital lobe sits beneath your parietal lobe, above your cerebellum. It is your vision centre. Sleep and brain health are bidirectional. You can support this relationship through the regulation of light, supporting eye health and engaging in meditation that strengthens the corpus callosum and regulates the circadian rhythm.

Ageing Eyes Impact Sleep

Macular degeneration is an eye disorder that affects the cells in the retina. As it advances, vision gets blurred and eventually leads to blindness. While it is age related, a major reason for it is inflammation of the eyes, oxidative stress and nutrient deficiencies.

I discovered a deep connection between ageing eyes, sleep and the health of the whole body during my research for this book. Ageing eyes increase light absorption and decrease pupil area, resulting in a progressive reduction of circadian receptivity. A ten-year-old has ten times greater reception to circadian impact as compared to a ninety-five-year-old. This can impact sleep and overall health, simply due to the degenerative health of the eyes.[8]

Recent research discovered specific cells in your retina that are triggered by light to then communicate with your brain and regulate your circadian rhythm and all its subsequent functions, including sleep.[9]

With ageing, the lenses of your eyes gradually turn yellow and the pupils become narrow. With these changes, less sunlight or daylight touches the eye and are unable to reach those cells in the retina that provide circadian feedback to the brain.[10]

What all this research proves is that it is critical to keep your eyes healthy and to delay their progressive ageing as it regulates and impacts the health of your full body via circadian rhythms.

4

The Circadian Rhythm

There is an amazing system within your body that connects your hypothalamus, pituitary and pineal glands. This system is what is called the circadian rhythm. It controls much more than just your sleep. Perhaps the earliest mention of a circadian rhythm can be found in Ayurveda. In recent years, there has been more concrete discoveries on this system. Jeffrey C. Hall, Michael Rosbash and Michael W. Young received the Nobel Prize in physiology or medicine for their discoveries of mechanisms controlling the circadian rhythm.[11]

Facts about the Circadian Rhythm

The circadian rhythm is a natural process that has been observed not just in humans but even in animals, plants, fungi and bacteria!

> **Did you know…**
>
> 1. Realigning a correct circadian rhythm can help your immune system calm down and relax.[12]

2. It is also crucial to your brain health. In fact, Dr Satchin Panda, who wrote *The Circadian Code*, points out that the circadian rhythm is present in almost all areas of your brain.
3. It regulates the health of your microbiome, digestion and liver health.[13] A good circadian rhythm helps your body prevent metabolic disorders such as diabetes and heart disease.
4. Waking up at dawn and doing mild exercises, stretches or yoga can have a positive impact on the overall circadian rhythm, and in turn restore your innate ability to have deep and healing sleep.[14]
5. Worshipping the sun is another way to help yourself. Get outside and do some sun salutations, swim when the sun is coming up, walk in the forest exposing yourself to the sun and play outside in the sun.
6. Circadian rhythms control eating as well. Your body is meant to eat a light breakfast, so that you have the support to work hard, a big lunch, which contains everything you require to support that hard work through the day, and a medium dinner not much past sunset, as digestion is weaker then.

When it comes to your circadian rhythm, just think back to the simple days of your ancestors. I remember my grandfather thinking that it was unheard of to wake up after the sun was up. Similarly, he would eat dinner around sunset or shortly after and then sit on his chair reading a book. He would not lounge around or lie down. Promptly after two hours, he would go to his bed and would be asleep in a few minutes. It was not the same for me over the years. At one point in time, my sleep was so bad that it would be a blessing if I slept one full night. I had to go back and learn many things to help me restore my sleep and I did, for the most part. Even today, if I do not fall back on some of these principles and practices which I talk about throughout this book, my sleep is impacted.

Can You Sneak in a Nap without It Impacting Your Natural Rhythm?

Napping is an area of confusion. There are so many different views on napping. The afternoon nap is often called a siesta and is integral to a relaxed lifestyle in many cultures, and perhaps a part of the weekend ritual.

I recall long ago that I prepared for a late night out by taking an afternoon nap so that my body could cope with staying awake. This is usually considered a prophylactic nap. I don't advice this anymore.

Short power naps in the afternoon have several benefits, including improvement of long-term memory,[15] vigour, alertness and cognitive performance.[16]

In general, research has not found afternoon naps to be detrimental. However, it is key that we look at ancient wisdom in this context, as someone struggling with sleep challenges or circadian misalignment might need to break that loop as well.

In Ayurveda, a lot of emphasis is placed on being in sync with nature. Afternoon naps are considered acceptable only for people who are usually unwell; therefore, it is meant as a recovery nap. It may also be acceptable in the peak of summer. Typically, the recommendation is to sleep in the afternoon for a short duration of twenty minutes, sitting upright, and before lunch—and only in these situations.

If you have several nights of poor sleep, one napping hack that works is to take a nap before lunch, rather than after. This allows you to recover without destroying your night's sleep.

> **Did you know ...**
>
> Often, people struggling with insomnia are suffering from what is referred to as a sleep-wake cycle disorder. This disorder is characterized by excessive daytime sleepiness, restless nights and frequent night-time awakenings. It is very common in shift workers, pilots, flight attendants and the elderly. Basically, in a sleep-wake cycle disorder, a person's circadian or daily rhythm is disturbed.
>
> To help reset the cycle, I recommend a special form of vitamin B12 known as methyl cobalamin. This can lead to improved sleep, increased daytime alertness, concentration and better mood.[17] Much of the benefit appears to be a result of methyl cobalamin influencing melatonin secretion.
>
> To help things even more, I also recommend taking melatonin about thirty minutes or so before bedtime. Melatonin has shown excellent results for both primary and secondary sleep disorders.[18] I have found using it in combination with methyl cobalamin makes it even more efficient. One month of methyl cobalamin in the morning and melatonin at bedtime should be plenty of time to reset your cycle.
>
> Michael T. Murray, N.D.
> Author, *The Longevity Matrix*
> www.DoctorMurray.com

Create a Ratricharya for Yourself: An Ayurvedic Nighttime Routine

Take yourself back to the time you were a child and you had a bedtime routine which involved getting into your pyjamas, brushing your teeth and curling up in your bed for a bedtime story!

1. Having an abhyanga before a bath is a great way to calm vata dosha and relax the nervous system. I go into this in more detail in the section on touch.
2. Eat a balanced dinner after a warm bath. It is ideal the meal is consumed before sunset.
3. Electric and magnetic fields from devices can impact sleep negatively. Consider setting a switch-off time for all devices. Set a window of three hours before bedtime with no exposure to blue light or mental stimulation. The section on the lights out challenge below by Sachin Patel will also go into how the right kind of light exposure can be beneficial.
4. Go to bed at the same time every day to set your circadian rhythm. Wake up at the same time every day, even during the weekend. It sounds simple, but it is easily overlooked. It is best to be in bed before 10 p.m. when pitta time of the night begins, which will then negatively impact sleep.
5. Make sure your sacred sleep space is different from the space where you watch television.
6. Replace TV or mobile phone usage with a habit that supports relaxation. Read a book which is calming and soothing to your brain.
7. Listen to guided meditations. People who meditate have higher levels of melatonin. We have several guided meditations on *The Sleep Whisperer Podcast*. Listen with an earpiece and eye mask for best results.

Lights Out Challenge

The lights out challenge is a three- to five-day challenge where we encourage participants to align their circadian rhythm with the rhythm of the sun. We awake prior to the sun to watch the sunrise and we align the rest of our day to fall with the setting of the sun—at which time we enjoy the sunset. If we can't enjoy the sunrise and sunset, then we at least synchronize rhythmically with the sun. Even on a cloudy day, going outside for a few minutes makes a big difference in your overall sense of well-being.

With the lights out challenge, our objective is to eliminate, as far as possible, artificial lighting and to decrease, minimize or eliminate exposure to lighting sources that are not naturally derived. This means that fire and candlelight, as well as very specific light bulbs that produce red light, can be used in the evening, as these have only an insignificant impact on melatonin. In fact, their impact, compared to the alternative, is negligible. Artificial light can reduce melatonin production by 60–80 per cent depending on the light bulb, thus leading to poor sleep, poor recovery, decreased immune function, fatigue, lack of cognitive function and all the other ill effects of poor sleep.

The lights out challenge is a good way to reset our rhythm with the rising and setting of the sun. During this challenge, it is also important to note the direction of your light source. During the day, the sun will be in the sky above us. The positioning of the sun sends important messages to our brain. When light is coming from above it hits the bottom of our retina, signalling to our brain that it is daytime, and so it is important that we stay alert and active. As the sun sets, our natural source of light for many thousands of years had been fire. This light hits the top of our retina, signalling to the brain that it's time to wind down. So, not only is the colour of light important, but also the angle. If you ever notice, a fire usually starts off burning yellow and then orange, and later turns into red embers before it goes out. This is the equivalent of the time after sunset, shifting our physiology from active recovery to preparation for deep sleep.

Oftentimes, we go from a state of overhead lighting that is bright and shining all day and right before we go to bed, at which time we turn it off completely. The challenge is simple. All I ask you to do is avoid artificial lighting as much as possible, turn off your computer screens and your phone as much as you possibly can, and switch to natural sources of lighting such as fire, candles or specific frequencies of red light using a flicker-free LED bulb.

Many of my clients have noticed radical shifts in their sleep and improvement in HRV (heart rate variability), and report feeling much calmer, waking up more energized and dreaming again, as well as having better mental clarity, focus and overall mood. The lights out challenge is, simply, a highly effective and cost-free way to significantly improve your health in a matter of days. I challenge you to turn the lights out.

Sachin Patel
Founder, Living Proof Institute

5

Your Inner Clock

Earlier, I spoke about the connection between Amara's eyes and her poor sleep. But did you catch what I said about her sleep and watching Netflix? This brings us to a critical aspect of sleep disruption, which is vata aggravation.

Vata dosha imbalance occurs when the eyes move rapidly, more so when stimulated by light, making the nervous system imbalanced and also impacting sleep. I talk about vata in detail in the section on sound.

How Facebook Taught Me about Light and My Inner Clock

More than a decade ago, I was first introduced to the world of social media by my husband. Today, he jokes to people about that introduction, for the first thing I said to him was, 'Who would want to waste their time on such useless things?' Fast forward to five years later: I had become addicted to Facebook and found myself caught in a routine where I stayed up, hidden under my blanket for fear of anyone disturbing my silent and secretive virtual world. Back then, I had a six-year-old who was fast asleep. I ignored my husband completely. My sleep was horrible.

As for what this was doing to my physiology, there were multiple things going on:

1. Firstly, I got a dopamine hit every time I checked Facebook.[19] Dopamine is an excitatory neurotransmitter hormone released in your brain which produces feelings of pleasure, alertness, concentration, euphoria and motivation. Yet, this kind of release, stimulated by the lights on a smartphone, is not a stable and sustained dopamine release, but a high. Afterwards, it leaves you with feelings of inadequacy, depression and dejection.
2. When light hits your retina, it is transmitted to your pineal gland, the area where serotonin is converted into melatonin. If light enters, then melatonin is suppressed[20] and cortisol is boosted.[21]

The Night Owl Phenomenon

There is evidence that genetics can determine whether you are a morning lark or a night owl. A small section of the population may indeed have those variations that make them a night owl.

Differing circadian rhythms that make someone a night owl or anything other than a morning lark may be a symptom or sign of several altered systems. We might be doing someone who thinks that they are a night owl an injustice by not digging deeper. Staying with this altered circadian rhythm and using it as a form of leverage to increase your productivity and work hours can be detrimental in the long run. My advice would be to first understand the potential root causes of your poor sleep. If you do want to look at genetics, consider testing. The right test for this is mentioned in the resources section of this book.

I disagree with the concept of altered sleep chronotypes except in some cases, and my personal view is that it can be the present state of imbalance that makes us night owls.

Do You Need Melatonin to Help You Sleep?

We are seeing more and more self-prescribed over-the-counter (OTC) melatonin, but is it required and is it safe? The answer to this is that it depends. Hold that thought for a moment and I'll come back to it.

Your pineal gland contains photoreceptors and is a light sensitive gland. It produces melatonin. As light decreases, melatonin increases and vice versa. It is the late evening release of melatonin that triggers a thermoregulatory effect and a subsequent decrease in core body temperature, which supports sleep.

There is an increase in core body temperature in the luteal phase of a menstrual cycle, which is the phase after ovulation. Some studies have found REM sleep to be reduced in this phase. It was also found that melatonin and progesterone influence each other.[22]

Typically, cortisol secretion happens in the morning to get us going and melatonin release occurs at night to help us sleep. When cortisol is elevated due to high stress, there is a natural decline in melatonin. It is advisable to look at all possible ways to reduce the heightened stress response and boost melatonin naturally before considering supplementation.

Melatonin is a powerful antioxidant, helping you deal with oxidative stress. When you take excessive non-steroidal anti-inflammatory drugs (NSAIDS), such as Ibuprofen, or large doses of B12 or similar shots, it can inhibit your release of melatonin, impacting not just your sleep, but also other aspects of health.[23] Caffeine and alcohol can also inhibit melatonin.

The best way to support melatonin is to begin living in harmony with nature's diurnal rhythms of light and dark before looking at supplementation. However, I have safely and effectively used melatonin in the process of weaning someone off sleeping pills. Therefore, it can have a place, but it is best done under supervision.

Gut health is at the core of all health. There is as much as 400 times more melatonin in a healthy gastrointestinal tract than even in the pineal glands. Melatonin release may influence gastrointestinal health directly through the central and autonomic nervous systems. It may also play a role in gut mucosal health, stomach acid secretion, epithelial health and circulation.[24]

Tricking the Pineal Gland with Different Lights

Can your pineal gland distinguish between natural and man-made light? Daylight has a duration. At one point, it gets dark and then your brain is programmed to prepare for sleep. The brain is also programmed to expect daylight on the retina during the day. Covering your eyes all day long also inhibits melatonin release.

6

Therapies for Your Sense of Sight

The ten-sense protocol at the end of the book brings together a structured plan, using tools and therapies from all the chapters. This chapter brings together different nutrients, protocols and therapies that you can utilize to help your eyes, circadian rhythm and sleep.

Vitamins and minerals for your eyes: Follow the basic supplement guide in the ten-sense protocol, and only add one targeted supplement for eye health and circadian support, if at all it is needed.* Consider your diet, lifestyle, stressors, routine and symptoms.

Melatonin supports the restoration of your circadian rhythm and brings you in sync with the earth's biorhythm. If you have not tried to dial in the changes necessary for improving your circadian

---

* Please also discuss with your doctor or health practitioner if you have any chronic health condition or if you are on any medication. Even though the protocol and supplements are researched and designed to work well for most people with sleep challenges, remember to stay aware and observe your own body for feedback, or work personally with your health practitioner. This is important if you are on any medication or if you are combining supplements.

rhythm, melatonin will not help you much. It is helpful to work with a practitioner when you want to wean yourself off sleeping medication.

Lutein is a wonder supplement for healthy eyes. It is a potent anti-inflammatory antioxidant. It can be found in egg yolks, leafy greens and orange fruits and vegetables. I can never forget the age-old advice to eat carrots for healthy eyes.

Blue light blockers: These have been my saving grace. If I must work staring at the computer screen all day, I wear them. In today's world, when you might possibly need to work looking at blue-light screens, I advise you to take the necessary precautions.

Turn on the night light on your gadgets towards sunset: If your device does not have this option, try using your device not too far beyond sunset, and if you do need to use it, then wear your blue light blockers.

Don't wear very dark sunglasses during the day: However stylish they may make you look, dark sunglasses aren't great for the day. When your retina is denied daylight, it struggles to set a healthy circadian rhythm. When you are outside, expose your eyes to natural light.

Therapies for Your Sense of Sight

In yogic wisdom, sadhana is considered a discipline of routine practice with an intention. Just as a seed takes time and nurturing to become a sapling to finally bearing fruit, anything in your body requires dedicated effort to bring about sustained change and reap benefits. Ayurveda and yoga have a wealth of knowledge when it comes to taking care of the senses. Think of sadhana as an ancient tradition with modern relevance.

Trataka

Trataka in yogic science means 'steady gaze'. It is deeply connected to the functioning of your pineal gland. Your eyes are connected to your pineal gland through your autonomic nervous system. The centre of your sympathetic and parasympathetic nervous system is the hypothalamus in your brain, which is also the centre for wakefulness and sleep. When you stare at an object until your eyes water profusely, it is a way of naturally cleansing your eyes without any external eye drops. It also brings about greater concentration and helps you move away from scattered thoughts. Trataka and crying cleanse the eyes.

How to Practice Trataka

1. Position a candle so the flame is at the same level as your eyes.
2. Sit comfortably and stare at the flame without blinking until your eyes water profusely.
3. When you cannot keep your eyes open any longer, close them and let your mind be still by concentrating on the image of the flame within your closed eyes.
4. After a minute, repeat the whole process again.

Try this practice for fifteen minutes daily. If you have any concerns but would like to add trataka into your daily life, you can always check with a trained yoga professional.

Eye Exercises

One of the things that I learnt at International Sivananda Yoga Vedanta Ashram at Neyyar Dam and Uttarkashi was how simple eye exercises were, yet how powerful they were to overall eye health and improved concentration. Simply add the following eye exercises to your routine, with ten repetitions each. Do them slowly, if possible, in sync with your breathing. Move your eyeballs:

1. Up and down
2. Side to side
3. Diagonally
4. Clockwise

Remember to do the above slowly. Relax your eyes between sets by gently cupping your palms over your eyes. Avoid slouching or moving your entire head. Ensure that you only use your eyes to move.

Sense Withdrawal to Soothe Your Eyes

In Ayurveda, sleep challenges can be associated with those who are predominantly vata dosha or anyone who has vata aggravation. When there is aggravation, the eyes tend to flicker and move constantly, which triggers an imbalance in the nervous system. Taking time to still the eyes can calm down vata dosha.

'Pratyahara' means 'sense withdrawal'. In the eight limbs of yoga, pratyahara is the fifth sense, referring to the practice of withdrawing your senses as a natural way to move your awareness, leading to a state of mental equilibrium.

Here are simple steps to practice pratyahara for your eyes:

1. To restrain your sense of sight, as a way to rest, gently close your eyes and lightly place your palms over them. Your palms should feel cool and it should be a very gentle touch.

2. After a minute, drop your palms.
3. Keep your eyes closed for a few minutes, while you observe the sensation within your closed eyes.

You can also try closing your eyes and applying some cool aloe vera gel over the eyelids for ten minutes. Wiping the eyelids with castor oil is helpful at night before sleep. Ayurveda offers several ways to care for the eyes. Keeping pitta in balance, which is discussed in the chapter on liver health, is key, since pitta dosha is related to the eyes. However, vata controls the movement of the eyes. Using one drop of ghee calms vata dosha and eye pressure. Traditional kajal used to highlight the eyes are made from soot and castor oil for this very purpose. You can also soak rose petals in water, dip a little bit of cotton or a piece of cloth in it and use this over eyelids.

How Amara Solved Her Sleep Problems

Amara started waking up and going to bed at fixed times. She made sure that she was asleep before 10 p.m. She took some time for herself each evening, practicing abhyanga and having a warm bath before dinner. She had dinner before sunset. After her meal, she put away her devices and gave her mind the space it needed to calm down. She made listening to guided meditation a night-time ritual. Before she went to sleep, she applied a drop of ghee to her eyes.

The Force that Governs How Well We Sleep

Getting a great night's sleep consistently, and waking up feeling refreshed and energized don't happen by chance. It happens by design. How well we sleep and how rested we feel when we wake up is governed by a universal code or rhythm. This code is called the circadian rhythm.

This rhythm exists in all animals, humans and plants.

How Plants Do It

Plants have light sensors that enable them to anticipate the sun's position in the sky, so that they can turn their leaves in the right direction throughout the day and harness solar energy for photosynthesis. Their leaves droop at night when the sun is down, and this enables plants to optimize energy intake and efficiency. What can we learn from plants?

Well, in order to optimize our energy and efficiency, we need to live in harmony with the law of rhythm by maximizing bright light during the day and soaking in complete darkness at night. Just like plants, we also have light sensors in the eyes, called melanopsin ganglion cells, that are designed to register the sun's position in the sky. Those sensors are most sensitive to blue light and much less sensitive to red light. When the sun is out, these light sensors are activated by registering the blue and green light, and they signal to our brain that it is daytime, maximizing energy production and enabling us to feel alert, focused and energized. In the absence of blue and green light, those light sensors signal to our brain that it is night-time, and our body starts preparing for sleep, healing and rejuvenation.

Blue Light Is Great During the Day

Early in the day, the sensitivity of light sensors (melanopsin) is low, which means we need a *lot* of light (1,00,000 lux or above) and, in particular, sunlight to set our clock mechanism. You might have heard that blue light is bad. This is only a half-truth because the reality is that you need blue light and a lot of it during the day to set your clock. It stimulates our brain more than any other colour, elevates our mood and increases our alertness. This is why most daytime blue light blockers are inefficient. In fact, blocking blue light during the day in the wrong way will cause circadian disruption and sleep problems.

Is Exposure to Blue Light from Screens and LED Bulbs Good for Me during the Day?

While blue light during the day is great, it can also be traffic. Are you wondering how? Well, think about it. The blue light you expose yourself to from sunlight is balanced and proportionate with all the other colours of the rainbow. In contrast, blue light coming from LED bulbs and screens peaks at 455 nm in blue-violet, which is deficient in the blue-turquoise, orange and red light that have regenerative properties, and thus very degenerative to our cells. Now, why did nature include a frequency that is degenerative? Well, this stimulating effect in nature increases free radical formation, just like exercise does. This causes mild and temporary oxidative stress. When this process is healthy and balanced, it regulates tissue growth and stimulates the production of antioxidants. What happens when we distort this balance through junk artificial light? Chronically being exposed to imbalanced blue artificial light will cause chronic oxidative stress, leading to cell and tissues damage as well as inflammation. This explains why overexposure to junk light during the day causes eye strain, headaches and agitation.

What's the Solution?

1. Download F.lux on your computer.
2. Wear high-quality daytime lenses like the ones Vivarays offer, which is designed to reduce the frequency of blue light at 455 nm, and make it more proportionate and balanced with the green and yellow light from the sun.
3. Take a five-minute sun break every two hours and expose your eyes to natural sunlight.

Blue Light Is Tragic at Night

The law of rhythm states that the day must become night. This means that high-frequency blue and green light will not be present in the environment. Your ability to live in harmony with this fact will determine to a great extent how healthy you are and how well you sleep.

While some people argue that blue light from artificial light sources at night is not bright enough to disrupt our circadian rhythm, the latest discovery in the field proves the opposite, which makes perfect sense because the circadian rhythm is governed by the universal law of rhythm.

Dr Samer Hattar is a senior investigator and chief of the section on light and circadian rhythms. He published a paper in *Cell*, showing how a little artificial light reaching the eyes at night suppresses the release of dopamine, the neuromodulator that makes us feel good and motivated. It also activates the habenula, also called the disappointment nucleus in the brain (thalamus) because it makes us feel less happy, and more disappointed and unsatisfied.

Why is it that very small amounts of light can be detrimental at night? Well, it's because our light sensors (melanopsin) become extremely sensitive to light at night, so much so that even a minute amount of artificial light at night will shift our circadian clock in the wrong direction and disturb our sleep.

Solution

1. Watch the sunset. When we do this, the melanopsin cells signal to the central clock that it is the end of the day. A study that was published showed that viewing the sunset adjusts our retinal sensitivity. This means that it will prevent some of the bad effects of artificial light in suppressing melatonin at night.
2. Wear high-quality lens technology after sunset, like Vivarays, which are designed to block all blue and green light and decrease brightness by twenty times, enabling your brain to understand that it is night-time while optimizing your melatonin production.
3. Place your night-time lighting low in the physical environment: Our melanopsin is located in the bottom half of the retina. We have a lens in front of our retina. Because of the nature of the optic of lenses, there is an

> inversion of the visual image. This means that those cells are most sensitive to overhead lighting.
>
> Roudy Nassif
> Cofounder of Vivarays

Create a Zen Zone that Is Soothing to Your Eyes

What can you do to support sleep using your vision? One way is to create a space which is soothing to your sense of sight. Allow your heart and soul to speak to you in choosing a room colour. Neutral colours which are soothing can be visual cues for your brain to prepare your body for sleep. Choosing lighter colours for bedding can be cosy, while dark colours can feel overwhelming. See that you have window dressing that keeps away light from the street and is as dark as is comfortable for you. You can choose to open them in the morning and have your eyes see sunlight coming into your room. If you read or want some light on for a while before you sleep, see that you use gentle lights.

PART 3

The Second Sense: Sound

7

Sound, Vata Dosha and Adrenals

What Do Ancient Wisdom and Modern Science Have to Say about Sound?

Ears symbolize memory, receptivity, the ability to listen, inquisitiveness and awakening. When it is gross, you hear. When it is subtle, you listen. You can use the subtle aspect consciously and reach a subtle state of spirit, which helps you to move into a parasympathetic nervous system response conducive to deep, restful and healing sleep.

You might not have any challenges with your ears, but your adrenals are more sensitive to sound than they are to any other sense stimuli. I will speak about adrenals in detail later. This connection is also correlated in Ayurveda. Vata dosha is responsible for the ears. Vata aggravation causes imbalance in the nervous system and to adrenal function.

How Sound Impacts Sleep

Tamara had various issues that didn't seem connected. Ten years ago, she had hurt her neck in a car accident and was asked to wear a neck brace to help her heal from the whiplash. She was only in her twenties then and did not think of looking any deeper into it. She wore the collar, her neck felt better and she moved on with her life. A few years later, however, she started to experience small episodes of dizziness. It first started in a yoga class, when she would feel dizzy each time she arched her back. She didn't think anything of it.

I asked her, 'Have you noticed any pattern to when you feel dizzy? Is it connected to any foods you eat, how you sleep, how stressed you are or any other pattern?'

She said that she felt uneasy in the car as well. Long drives made her feel nauseous and dizzy. When it was bad, it triggered episodes of vertigo as well. She felt the room was spinning and if she looked up or down, everything felt strange.

I asked her, 'What do you think prevents you from having deep sleep? Do you struggle with any pain in your neck? Can you pinpoint what is the biggest reason you don't fall asleep?'

She replied, 'In the last few months, I've developed a symptom which is very scary and overwhelming. I have ringing in my ears. Sometimes it starts as I am about to fall asleep, and I feel anxiety and sometimes have panic attacks. It makes me stress so much that I then cannot fall asleep.'

I also asked about how she coped with stress. She said she had frequent episodes of panic and fear, was overwhelmed a great deal and found the smallest of stressors making her very jumpy for days afterwards. She did not express herself to anyone.

Understanding the Ears and Your Sense of Sound

Tamara experiences dizziness, balance issues, vertigo and ringing in her ears. All these contributed to how sensitive she was to sound. Years of excessive stress had set her autonomic nervous system in fight-or-flight mode. Sound triggered severe stress, which made her lose sleep for days. The adrenals impact sleep greatly and are especially sensitive to disruption through sound more than any other sense.

From an Ayurvedic perspective, this high stress led to imbalanced vata dosha in Tamara.

Excess Vata Dosha Causes Sleep Deficiency

Looking from the perspective of Ayurveda helps us understand this connection between sound, adrenal function, the nervous system and sleep. We do not have the space to explore Ayurveda and the doshas in detail, but I'll share some main aspects which will bring this chapter together for you.

Ayurveda speaks about disease having three primary causes, which are suppressing natural urges, misusing the senses and the effect of seasonal shifts. We can misuse our senses by underusing, overusing or misusing them.

Vata, pitta and kapha are the three doshas within our body. Dosha can be described in several ways. All three doshas move in our body in unique combinations that then decide our constitution. Their unique combination at birth is our Prakriti. Their provoked or imbalanced state is our Vikriti. How the three come together in unique ways at birth decides our body structure, hair colour, eye colour, digestive patterns, emotional tendencies and temperament towards specific diseases.

Vata is responsible for the movement in the body. The qualities of vata are cold, light, airy, dry, subtle, mobile, sharp, flowing, hard, rough and clear. It governs our mind, senses, nervous system, balance, motor organs and adrenal function.

Because it has a mobile quality, moving the eyes quickly can imbalance vata. Disturbing sounds can also imbalance vata as the ears are a home to vata.

The functions of vata are too many to discuss here. Some include the energy of respiration, nerve impulse, state of mind, circulation and the vibration that becomes the heartbeat. Vata affects the mind and body via the nervous system.

The primary home of vata dosha is in the colon. Additional homes of vata include the ears, thighs, hips, bones, hearing and touch. Even though the eyes are the not home to vata, the movement in the eyes is controlled by vata and rapid movement disrupts it.

Due to its mobile nature, vata easily goes off balance. Triggers of vata imbalance include stimulation through scrolling, dehydration, dry foods, excess heat, multitasking, travel, over exercising, too much talking, a disrupted circadian rhythm, dryness, lack of sleep, medication and stimulants.

Other symptoms of vata aggravation include weakness, an aversion to cold, feeling cold, pain, numbness, digestive problems, erratic digestion, constipation, insecurity, fear, anxiety, dizziness, premenstrual syndrome (PMS), dehydration, palpitations, increased heart rate, restlessness, scattered mind, frequent urination, shallow breathing and a tendency towards addictions. Much of this is linked to the inability to fall asleep.

Someone who is predominantly vata dosha, or someone who has vata aggravation, can be a light sleeper, toss and turn and wake up for no reason. Their ability to sleep varies night to night, and they may frequently sleepwalk and sleep talk. Ringing in the ears is a sign of vata aggravation as well.

Caring for the ears and hearing is associated with calming vata dosha and relaxing the nervous system. Covering the ears while sleeping keeps vata calm. I have mentioned the practice of karna purana at the end of this chapter. Caring for the ears includes karna purana and marma pressure points. Marmas are vital points in the body in Ayurvedic anatomy. They are usually located over lymph nodes, where veins, tendons, joints, muscles and bones come together. They are important in treating any condition. They can be treated with pressure, warmth, herbal oils and massage. There are marma points that help with the ears. Karna moola is the marma just below the ears. Viduram is a marma point at the base of the skull on either side of the spine. All head marmas calm the five vayus and vata dosha. Please consult an expert if you are interested in marmas. Keeping vata balanced can help improve sleep tremendously.

The Environment of Your Ears

If your microbiome is not a healthy one, then you could have more pathogenic bacteria in the middle ear. When excess vata dries up the ear, there will be a tendency for irritation, build-up of wax or for water to get stuck easily.

Relax Your Neck to Help You Sleep

It can really help the health of your ears to have structural movement and exercise developed for healthy blood circulation in your neck. Spinal misalignments at the neck can impact systems within the body. Vata is said to enter at the back of the neck. In Ayurveda, the practice of covering the neck while walking outdoors is to prevent imbalance in vata dosha. Neck pain is a sign of vata aggravation.

> This fascinating connection can help you in many ways:
>
> 1. When you have recurrent ear issues, there will be some localized inflammation in the middle ear and a build-up of fluid. Fluid that gets trapped within your middle ears becomes a ripe breeding ground for infections. Relaxing the neck and improving blood flow around the eustachian tubes can help proper drainage.
> 2. If you practice yoga, then simple neck exercises with breath coordination and postures, like shoulder stand and fish, can be beneficial. If you have spondylitis, then shoulder stand is contraindicated. If so, stay with fish pose and gentle twists, which move your neck to each side.
> 3. My practice to relax the neck is a warm sesame oil massage, right from the nape of the neck to the tip of my toes. I allow the oil to soak for fifteen minutes. I go into this practice in full detail in the section on abhyanga in the chapter on touch. Nothing else has helped my chronic neck pain as much as regular abhyanga.

Can Ringing in the Ears Be Calmed Down?

Autoimmunity is becoming more and more common today, and women are at especially high risk.[25] This is probably because a woman's immune system is flexible, allowing a foetus to grow, even though it typically does not belong to her body, has chromosomal differences and hormone fluctuations.

Ringing in the ears is also known as tinnitus. 'Tinnitus' comes from a Latin word which means 'to ring'. It can also refer to hearing sounds differently or abnormally.

Ringing in the ears and anxiety are both symptoms of excess vata.

Reasons for ringing in the ears include any kind of nerve damage or eardrum rupture, which can easily happen on a flight or due to stress, smoking, anxiety, tension in the neck, toxic exposure, loud sounds, frequent colds, build-up of earwax, some types of medication, anaemia, dehydration, fluctuating blood pressure, food sensitivities, gut issues, excess vata and nervous system imbalance. *I would reiterate that keeping vata balanced is the most powerful tool for you.*

Tinnitus is just one symptom of vata imbalance. It lets you know that vata has to be calmed down. I know that we all tend to worry about a symptom, but what we if consider that these provide us with a tool for understanding our body? When we have symptoms like ringing in the ears, strive for a deeper understanding of vata dosha. Look at the triggers of vata imbalance so you can create a list of what might be the cause in your case. After eliminating the triggers, use vata calming tools to help your body. Reframe your mind from feeling fear over one symptom to using the fear to understand your body as a whole.

8

Adrenal Function, the HPA Axis and Sound

What Do Your Adrenal Glands Do?

I had no idea that I had adrenal glands until thirteen years ago, when my son was born with an adrenal disorder. Little did I know how much power they exerted over our overall well-being.

The adrenal glands sit on top of your kidneys, which is why the name 'ad renal'. The adrenal glands have an outer layer called the cortex and an inner layer called the medulla. The cortex produces cortisol, aldosterone and androgens. The medulla produces norepinephrine, epinephrine and dopamine.

Cortisol is a critical hormone. It plays many roles, including that of regulating blood sugar, increasing blood pressure, modulating inflammation, increasing appetite and energy levels, and taming allergies. If you have dysfunctional cortisol rhythms, then you can have poor appetite, low energy, low blood pressure and low blood sugar. Cortisol has a particular biorhythm. It is supposed to be highest at the start of your day and lowest when you fall asleep.[26]

The cortex also produces testosterone and dehydroisoandrosterone (DHEA), which is the precursor to testosterone, as well as oestrogen and progesterone. Epinephrine, which you might know as adrenaline, is the fight-or-flight response. Norepinephrine is a neurotransmitter, while dopamine is a neurotransmitter related to feeling pleasure, alertness, concentration, euphoria and motivation.

Aldosterone regulates the balance of sodium potassium in your blood and urine, and of salt and water in your system. Compromised function can also lead to symptoms such as excessive thirst, raising pulse, light-headedness, dizziness, fatigue, craving salty food and frequent urination. Many of these are symptoms of excess vata!

Are you confused here? I was! The fact is that the adrenal glands are a backup system for your sex hormones.[27]

How Tamara Experienced Adrenal Issues

So, what happens in your body during different phases of adrenal dysfunction? For the longest time, Tamara assumed she could not sleep because she had too much energy. She used to feel a buzz in her body and a racing pulse. She could never sleep, however exhausted she was. After years of being in a marriage which caused severe stress, she was perpetually in a state of fight or flight. She could not wind down, even when she was out of the situation.[28]

Tamara started to have digestive problems, irrational hunger, cravings and water retention—so much so that at times she could not wear regular clothes. She experienced low blood pressure and a completely messed up sleep cycle. She had fatigue so severe that she would wake up feeling heavy gloom and depression. When Tamara came out of the marriage, she found herself struggling with the other extreme of feeling exhausted no matter how much rest she got. It was as though her adrenals were telling her that they had had enough of the onslaught of stress.

What Adrenal Dysfunction Looks Like

There is a connected system between your hypothalamus, pituitary and adrenal glands, which is called the HPA axis. In stress, your hypothalamus secretes a hormone called corticotropin releasing hormone (CRH). It triggers your pituitary to release adrenocorticotropic hormone (ACTH), which travels to your adrenal cortex and triggers the release of cortisol.

Cortisol has a specific biorhythm; your body has been set to a specific wave. If you break that sync, you will have adrenal fluctuations. The body is complex, especially the endocrine systems, and there are deep feedback loops in place between the brain and different glands. In the case of the adrenal glands, this function is performed by the HPA axis. Actual cortisol production takes place in the adrenal glands, but the brain controls the circadian rhythm and how, how much and when cortisol should be released.[29]

Adrenal function can be compromised by so many things; anything from trauma in the brain, constant exposure to stress and the inability to find ways to cope, low-fat diets, skipping meals, constant low blood pressure, low-salt diets, over exercise, under-sleeping and stress can affect it. Inner balance is key. Some of these are also triggers of vata imbalance. The first step must be to reduce these triggers. Tamara would place stress and poor sleep as the highest triggers of these. She had to stay awake through the night for many years, for that was the only way she could protect herself from an alcoholic spouse. Stress is not bad. It is a natural response. Constant stress is bad. In this case, the stress response does not shut off and resilience to stress starts to reduce.

The Impact of Sound on Your Adrenals

I'll share another story about Tamara before I take you through the research on the impact of sound on the adrenal system. In her stressful marriage, Tamara's brain had programmed itself to a particular sound. It was the sound of a cupboard door opening in the middle of the night, which indicated to her that her ex-husband had come home. She did not think anything of it, but many years later, when she remarried, she was alarmed at an incident that occurred.

One night, Tamara was sleepy and went to bed. Her husband stayed awake to watch a little television and when he went to bed later, he opened the cupboard door to change his clothes. Tamara was fast asleep, but somewhere deep in her brain, that sound triggered a chain of events. She said she woke up panting and sweating profusely, and sat up in bed, completely disoriented. Her husband was alarmed by this reaction, but quickly realized that there was a connection to her past story. He hurried over to her, hugged her tight and reassured her. She slowly relaxed to the point where she was no longer disoriented, but it took her a while to fall back asleep. When I asked her about incidents that triggered panic, she recalled this as one which had made a deep impact on her, though she had not understood why.

Recently, I went to a party which went on for most of the night. This is not something I do all the time. The music was extremely loud, as is the case in most events today. I was also driving past a car which was blaring music so loudly that my son said he felt the reverberations in our car and on the road. Sound pollution has been found to increase the stress hormone cortisol and may be related to the effect of noise on your HPA axis.[30] Your sound system is permanently open, even in your sleep! Noise signals are deeply connected via your amygdala to your HPA axis.

The amygdala is an area in your brain which wants you to stay as you are. Noise was found to cause a release on the whole cascade of stress hormones via the HPA axis. A few days after this all-night party with blaring music, I found myself unable to sleep after a long time. When I lay down, my cortisol spiked and I found myself wide awake.

Loud sounds increase the secretion of corticotrophin, which then causes an increase in cortisol. Higher ACTH can also cause an increase in aldosterone. Can you make some connections in your mind? Dysfunctional aldosterone, that key hormone which regulates sodium and potassium, can cause electrolyte issues, resulting in dizziness, thirst, craving salt, frequent urination, raising pulse and feeling light-headed.[31] Many of these links back to vata excess.

Do you see how many connections there are to sound and adrenals? Beyond most of your senses, your adrenals are particularly sensitive to sound.

Adrenal glands can be impacted if there is an excess of stimulation or inadequate nourishment. It can also be impacted by personalities who are what is called 'Type A'—always wanting to overachieve, for whom nothing is ever enough. This is what someone who is vata predominant or imbalanced in vata may tend to do. The yogic belief is that if you take anything to an extreme, like overusing your adrenal glands and the stress response, you've already set the opposite effect in motion: Burnout.

Create a Healing Routine to Calm Vata Dosha and Stabilize Adrenal Function

Let me break up this whole chapter into easy-to-apply steps to restore adrenal balance. When it comes to this aspect:

1. **Avoid aggravating vata**, be it from excess stimulants like alcohol, caffeine and sugar, or be it from excessive exercise. Overall, vata can be calmed down with warm sesame oil abhyanga, which is mentioned in detail in the chapter on touch, being in harmony with nature's circadian rhythm, warm and moist food, reduced overactivity and stimulation, and daily meditation. All these are also associated with better sleep. My favourite vata calming practice is to lie on the ground on a carpet, place a silk eye mask with a drop of sweet orange essential oil on it over my eyelids and listen to one of the guided meditations on *The Sleep Whisperer Podcast* with earphones. It is helpful to reduce heavier legumes like kidney beans for some time until agni is strong. Restrict heavier legumes to lunch, when agni is naturally high, and keep lighter legumes like mung for dinner. This does not mean they should never be consumed. Potatoes are best avoided at all times. Vata needs adequate healthy fats, especially from ghee. A low-fat diet can trigger vata imbalance. When you are outside, if there is a strong wind, cover yourself well, especially the back of the neck and ears.
2. **Restore your circadian rhythm**. Your adrenal glands cannot cope with unnatural rhythms for long. A disrupted circadian rhythm is a trigger of vata imbalance.
3. **Balance blood sugar**. Without balancing blood sugar, you cannot have a regulated stress response.

4. **Avoid constipation** as it can increase adrenal issues and allow cortisol to stay in your body.[32] The chapter on detoxification will take you through this aspect in depth. Constipation is a sign of increased vata dosha. It is a sign that the system is too dry.
5. **Eliminate caffeine** even if you hear that you can safely consume it during the day. Caffeine prevents cortisol from coming down at night when you need to sleep.[33] Caffeine can increase anxiety in excess vata, dries out the digestive tract and leads to an overwrought nervous system.
6. **Avoid any restrictive diets.** Missing meals and restrictive diets can make your adrenals unstable. Skipping meals aggravates vata dosha.

9

Therapies for Your Sense of Sound

Using Sound to Soothe Your Adrenals

When it comes to your sense of hearing, you can be magically transported into a world of imagination and healing, through music and meditation.

Are there sounds which are sweet and pleasing in your life? Is there music that might bring back memories or remind you of the gentle voice of someone who loves you dearly? Listening can be the magical medium of peace. Bring in soothing sounds into your life every day.

Begin by removing the sounds of electronic gadgets, whether it is the sound of TV shows that are exciting and stimulating and the sounds of notifications on the phone, which can trigger your brain to be focused on the external world. It does take dedication to stay away from gadgets for a minimum of two hours before you sleep, where you cannot hear your phone at all. It is best to use an old-fashioned alarm clock to wake up. Silence your phone altogether before bedtime.

Replenish Micronutrients for Your Ears and Adrenal Support

No supplement can outsmart an unhealthy diet and lifestyle. Remember that you cannot take all the supplements that exist. Please consider the specific nutrients mentioned in the chapters here only after you have tried the basic recommendations in the protocol. Please also discuss with your doctor or health practitioner if you have any chronic health condition or if you are on any medication.

L-Theanine

L-theanine is a compound found in green tea, which has a calming effect on your brain. It is thought to cross the blood brain barrier easily, where it reaches your brain and positively affects amino acid levels, therefore influencing serotonin and other neurotransmitters.

Ashwagandha

Ashwagandha has been the gem of Ayurveda for time immemorial. Considered a miracle for dealing with the impact of stress on your body and your mind, ashwagandha is an adaptogenic herb. It supports your body and calms vata dosha, but you need to exercise caution if you have inflammatory conditions and are sensitive to nightshades.

Therapies for Your Sense of Sound

Sound has been used since ancient times to bring about profound change. From chanting to humming, it is utilized to lighten the mind and uplift the spirit. Think about why you feel so much better when you walk in the park or bathe in the woods. Sounds from ancient therapies can be rooting and anchoring. The adrenal glands are the root of so many other systems, and sound can become that powerful force in building this safe scaffolding for you. This is a foundational principle of guided meditation. There are so many wonderful therapies to support your adrenals through sound. Try them!

Brahmari Pranayama

Brahmari is known as the humming bee breath in yogic wisdom. It is a wonderfully simple practice that can be done even by children. The sound of humming within the brain is immensely tranquil and calming. Brahmari releases cerebral tension as well. It reduces anger, which can be a big part of adrenal issues. It releases anxiety and strengthens the throat. Since the ear, nose and throat are all connected, brahmari is a wonderful practice to add as sadhana for your sense of sound. It calms down vata dosha.

Here are the simple steps to practising brahmari pranayama:

1. It is helpful to practise brahmari at night before you sleep. Sit up in bed, leaning back comfortably. Close your eyes and relax your whole body. Your lips should be gently closed with your teeth slightly separated.
2. Raise the arms up and ball them into fists. Use your thumbs to close the flap of each ear and seal off external sound.
3. Inhale through your nostrils. Breathe out very slowly, making a deep steady humming sound. The sound should be smooth and not jerky. It should be mellow and soft and soothing, allowing you to feel the gentle vibration within the skull.

4. Do five to ten rounds at first, and then increase it to fifteen minutes.

If you have severe stress, stay with fifteen minutes of this soothing practice. Set an intention that you are using this sadhana for your sense of sound, to restore balanced adrenals and support deep sleep. Humming also increases nitric oxide production.[34] I talk about this more in the section on smell.

Baoding Balls

Many years ago, a friend of mine went to Tibet and got me some Tibetan stress balls. I loved them and still use them. I close my eyes and gently move them near my ears. The sound of the distant chiming is magical and soothing. In fact, research found that 'listening to Tibetan music could help patients to manage preoperative anxiety. The implementation of music is easy to administer, and should be considered for clinical practice'[35]

Music as Sound Energy

Talking about music, I come from a culture where all children learn music, either classical singing or an instrument. Even today, when I listen to classical music or listen to a magical instrument like the flute, I find myself with tears in my eyes and in a divine space of mind.

I also want to speak about research when it comes to music. In research on women with breast cancer, it was found that a single session of music targeted at those who have a higher level of sympathetic tone activity was effective in reducing many symptom clusters. This points us back to the fact that the adrenals are at the root of healing. To heal from any complex health challenge, you are required to move into a parasympathetic nervous system response, where you can rest, digest and heal.[36]

Karna Purana

Karna purana is an ancient Ayurvedic practice to take care of the ears and calm down vata dosha. While I explain the practice here, I also suggest going to a skilled practitioner who can do this for you, based on your individual constitution, state of imbalance and any other concerns.

1. It is ideal to lay a plastic sheet on the floor with an old towel on it. Layer some old paper where your head will be.
2. Lie down on one side and gently start filling warm sesame oil into the ear that is exposed. Use a dropper to add it slowly.
3. Allow the warm oil to trickle into the ear canal for five to twenty minutes or based on the advice of your practitioner.
4. Afterwards, turn over and repeat the same procedure on the other ear, during which time the oil from the first ear will ooze out.

This practice combats excess dryness within the ear, calms vata dosha and balances the nervous system. It should only be done once every few months, unless otherwise advised.

Sense Withdrawal to Soothe Your Ears

To restrain your sense of sound, listen to the sound of silence for a few minutes daily. This can be challenging. First, start to become mindful of whether you seem to need sound all the time. Is the silence difficult for you to handle? Sit for a few minutes, perhaps after your brahmari, and just listen to the sound of silence. Think of silence as that gap or pause between any two sounds. Try and hear silence well. After a few days of this practice, you'll find that you can tune in to the sound of silence much more easily than before. Alternatively, listen to the sound of your own breath for a while. Slowly, soften your breath more and more, until your breath is slow, soft, silent and subtle. This will lead you into the sound of silence, where you can stay for a few minutes to rest your sense of sound and give it space to recover. Try to practice sitting for five minutes without interruption one to three times daily. Set a timer and quieten your mind.

How Tamara Solved Her Sleep Problems

Tamara started to calm her vata by learning to do less, not feeling pressured by a to-do list and teaching herself to say no. She took ten minutes every afternoon to lie down on the floor and listen to a soothing guided meditation. She scheduled this into her calendar so that it became a habit. She used to convince herself that a little coffee in the morning was not impacting her sleep by searching for health experts who spoke in favour of having it in the morning. As a test, she weaned herself off coffee and noticed her anxiety coming down. Each night in bed, she practised ten minutes of brahmari. She was pleasantly surprised by how these simple interventions, which did not take too much of her day, transformed her sleep.

PART 4

The Third Sense: Smell

10

Smell, Emotions and Memories

Your sense of smell is associated with the element of earth. Smell is deeply linked to memories. If you smell and taste food that connects you to a loving ancestor, you can go to sleep with feelings of safety and peace. Smell influences the limbic brain, and can influence how you react to stress and fear.

Ayurveda and the Glymphatic System

Recently, researchers defined a system in the human body which they called the glymphatic system, which is a system that removes waste and detoxifies the brain, a discovery that could make a world of difference for neurological conditions.

The glymphatic system is a waste clearance system that uses a unique vascular system for efficient elimination of metabolites from the central nervous system. This system is also used for distribution of glucose, lipids, amino acids, growth factors and neuromodulators through the brain. When there is inflammation in the brain, glial cells are inflamed, causing restrictions to the flow of cerebral spinal fluid. This starts to impact how neurons are fired and how the brain starts to decline. The waste that accumulates from inflamed glial cells is called beta amyloid plaque.

Why is the healthy functioning of your glymphatic system crucial? Glymph is a waste clearance pathway to remove excess protein and metabolites from the brain and spinal cord. Waste clearance happens only in deep sleep.[37] Glymph that is not cleared has been linked to mental health challenges, from brain fog and anxiety to depression and more serious mental illness. This glymphatic system was understood in Ayurveda to be connected to some body constitutions that are predisposed towards sinus challenges and mental health symptoms.

Is Smell Linked to Poor Sleep?

Tara was in her late thirties and was constantly struggling with colds, sinus attacks, headaches and severe congestion. She could not get through the day without nose drops. It helped her only for a few hours and then her nose was stuffy again. She had headaches and fatigue and ended up breathing through her mouth at night due to disturbed sleep. She had tried many things, but only found temporary relief. Her nose drops were opioids; she knew they might have side effects and was keen to get off them. She was open to change, but felt she was at rock bottom.

She said that she slept for eight to nine hours, but her sleep was broken by episodes where she woke up, unable to breathe. She would keep moving to find a position that would support her breathing. Her broken sleep made her feel tired in the morning and her head felt heavy. She relied on cheese as a major source of protein. Her system was getting congested with heavy foods, not allowing her to feel light. She waited for her partner to come home before eating dinner at 9 p.m. She then ate a cheese sandwich or some pasta. She went to sleep within about half an hour of eating.

Nose, Smell, Kapha Dosha, Sleep Apnoea and Sleep

Ayurveda connects concepts that do not appear to have an outward relation to each other. In Ayurveda, kapha dosha relates to the nose, head and the sense of smell. Kapha gives stability to the body and holds everything together. The qualities of kapha dosha are cold, heavy, wet, gross, dense, static, dull, soft, smooth, cloudy and white. It is responsible for nourishment, support, the bulk of tissues and aspects of the mind such as the ability to be compassionate.

Some of the functions of kapha include the forming of the skeleton, muscles, organs, ligaments, tendons and the skin. Kapha holds our joints together. It is also responsible for the thin layer of fat around the organs.

The primary home of kapha dosha is in the stomach. Additional homes of kapha are the chest, throat, head, pancreas, lymph, fat, nose and mouth.

Triggers of kapha imbalance include heavy food, dairy, sugar, starch, a sedentary lifestyle, lack of movement and sleeping past sunset.

Symptoms of kapha aggravation include depression, lethargy, stagnation, obesity, aversion to cold, sticky mucus, sleep apnoea, wet cough, cloudy urine, excess salivation, repeated chest congestion, sluggish digestion, bloating, difficulty breathing, allergies and cravings.

Someone who is predominantly kapha dosha or who has kapha aggravation might sleep easily but heavily, may sleep longer than advised and can wake up with a gasp. They may have sleep apnoea or a tendency for mouth breathing.

Overall, kapha can be calmed down by avoiding congesting foods like dairy, taking regular walks or exercising daily, including warming spices such as turmeric, cinnamon and black pepper in the diet, avoiding heavy food, eating lighter food and eliminating sugar, practising pranayama for proper breathing and incorporating a dynamic yoga practice such as vinyasa.

Caring for the nose and smell is associated with better breathing. These practices are mentioned at the end of this chapter and include the practice of jal neti and nasyam every day. This allows the maintenance of a healthy nasal system. There are marma points which support caring for the nose. These pressure points are at the centre of and above the eyebrows. Keeping kapha balanced helps to reduce symptoms of sleep apnoea and prevent mouth breathing, as well as increasing the feeling of being grounded and improves longevity.

Is Your Stuffy Nose a Sign of Deeper Challenges?

It's scary how many people suffer from sinusitis today. Like Tara, there are thousands of people suffering every single day. Here, I provide some information about your sinus to get you started.

A sinus infection, also known as sinusitis, is a very common upper respiratory tract infection that occurs when your nasal cavities are swollen and inflamed. You can suffer from severe pain in your face, especially around your nose, in your upper jaw, between your eyes, under your eyes and in your head. Mucosa associated lymphoid tissue, or MALT, is a concentration of lymph tissue in all the areas where you have mucosa or wet tissue. This is found within your respiratory system, including your nasal cavity.

Kapha body constitutions or kapha imbalance can lean towards dysbiosis and sinus issues.

When your mucous membranes get inflamed, then it can block the nasal passage and prevent fluid draining in the sinus, causing the fluid to remain there and breed bacteria, leading to more infection.

Environmental toxins play a big role on your health. You are surrounded by toxins, from cigarette smoke to pollution to mould. Practices like jal neti can help counter their effects.

Nutrient deficiencies could also be at the root of your sinusitis. Micronutrient deficiencies are closely intertwined with poor digestive health and weak agni.

Jal neti is a great tool for healthy mucous secretion in the nasal cavity. It can help balance secretion, humidify the mucosa, disrupt any biofilm of pathogenic bacteria and flush out pathogens. Jal neti is wonderfully supportive only when practised continuously. Attempting to do so sporadically whenever you feel congested is risky and ineffective.

You Could Get Hooked to Nasal Sprays

Most nasal sprays are meant to be used just for a few days. In reality, they end up being used for a long term, leading to nasal spray addictions. One study found half of its participants were long-term nasal spray users and were in a state of addiction. While it is not an addiction in the true sense of the word, the fact is that they can cause tissue damage in the mucosa, leading to swelling and long-term stuffiness.[38]

If you've been using any decongestant nasal sprays, then you need to be cautious of the impact of long-term use, which can also include, as with many nasal sprays, rebound congestion, which is when you are unable to go on without using the spray. Do you ever feel that you get more congested each time you try to withdraw your usage? Do you find that you are still using your spray, but just not getting the relief you require?

Remove your dependence to them by topping your nasal spray with water each time you use a few drops. This ensures that the bottle stays full always. Over time, it starts diluting the opioid spray slowly. It takes several months, but, eventually, you train yourself to not need it without having to face strong rebound reactions. Please do so under the guidance of a doctor or a health practitioner.

11

Breath: The Symbol of Prana

Ancient Wisdom Got Breath Perfectly Right

Globally, there is much emphasis on the importance of breath in all health. I would just like to bring your attention to what are some of the most important points to observe in yourself. Breathing occurs most often without conscious thought or awareness. Over time, there has been a suboptimal shift in breathing patterns in many of us.

There is a saying in yoga that we have a specific number of breaths. The slower we breathe, the longer we are supposed to live.

When you are in a sympathetic dominant state, a fight-or-flight state in high stress, then your body releases adrenaline—pupils dilate, blood vessels constrict, digestion stops, heart rate and body temperature increase, immune function weakens and reproductive function reduces. All these can be associated with poor sleep, high stress and, therefore, reduction in the quality of health. Breath is critical. In a parasympathetic state, when you consciously slow down breathing, you also help your body release acetylcholine, your pupils constrict, heart rate and temperature decrease, and your immune function and hormones are boosted, all of which support sleep.

Breathing patterns and where you breathe from play a key role as well. For this, it is important to go into the physiology of the breath. To understand that, you need to look at the lungs and the diaphragm. Your lungs are two bags that can be inflated and deflated. They are surrounded on the sides by your ribcage. Below them is an important muscle called the diaphragm. When you consciously expand your abdomen, your diaphragm moves down, creating a vacuum in the chest that allows your lungs to fill with air. Relaxation of the abdominal muscles then reduces the volume of air in your chest and allows you to exhale. Breathing by using your diaphragm allows you take in the greatest amount of air, as compared to a shallow breath, which occurs when you expand your ribcage without using the diaphragm. It is important to note that abdominal breathing helps you shift into a parasympathetic state. It also provides a gentle massage to the organs within the abdominal cavity, including the liver, and increases oxygenation within your body. Since breathing, unlike respiration, is both involuntary and voluntary, we have great power in our hands with our breath.

Never Ignore Your Tendency towards Mouth Breathing

Breathing through your nose and mouth are very different. Observe anyone who has challenges with physical or emotional health when they sleep, and you might notice that they sleep with their mouth open. Mouth breathing activates the sympathetic nervous system. It also reduces nitric oxide, and impacts the lymphatic and circulatory systems. Nasal breathing activates the parasympathetic nervous system, increases nitric oxide production, improves lymphatic movement and helps build resilience to stress.

Retraining Yourself to Breathe Right

While I have included some practices throughout this book, here, let's look at the simplest way to breathe well, which is using the diaphragm and breathing through your nose.

How to breathe effectively to calm down:

1. Sit comfortably. Place one palm on your abdomen to guide you.
2. When you inhale, gently feel your abdomen moving outwards and gently push your palm to ensure that you use the diaphragm and not the ribcage.
3. When you exhale, use your palm to gently guide your abdomen to relax, allowing your diaphragm to lift upwards and release air. Try to ensure that your ribcage does not move when you do this and make sure that you do not breathe through your mouth.
4. With every breath, try and slow it down ever so slightly. You could also count to four when you inhale and to eight when you exhale if that feels comfortable and relaxing. The longer your exhalation is in comparison to the inhalation, the better your vagal tone, which is your ability to balance the autonomic nervous system.

Even doing this for ten minutes a day will help your whole physiology shift. You can find several guided breath sessions on my podcast. I mention this in the Resources as well.

Nasal breathing helps to activate the parasympathetic nervous system, allows your heart rate to slow down, creates a drop in temperature and supports better sleep.

12

The Glymphatic System and Sleep

The glymph is a waste clearance pathway for excess protein and metabolites from the brain and spinal cord. This process happens only in deep sleep. Your lymphatic and glymphatic systems are interconnected. Understanding kapha dosha makes this clear.

The glymphatic system is most active when you are in deep sleep, and is implicated in every form of neuroinflammation and degeneration—from sinusitis to depression to the development of more complex neurodegenerative conditions like Alzheimer's and Parkinson's. The glymphatic system gets its name from glial cells and the lymphatic system. One of the most critical factors affecting the functioning of this system is interstitial space volume, which is said to increase when you are in deep sleep.[39]

Quality of sleep and exercise are considered crucial to how efficiently your glymphatic system works. Ensuring that you walk 10,000 steps daily can be helpful to the lymphatic and glymphatic systems. Why not incorporate some wonderful ancient tools into your daily life?

What Is the Limbic Brain and How Is It Connected to Smell and Sleep?

In your brain, the cerebrum has right and left hemispheres, held together by the corpus callosum, which helps these two hemispheres communicate with each other. The cerebrum is your forebrain and is the most superior part of your entire nervous system. It occupies the whole upper part of your skull.

I only mentioned the cerebrum for you to visualize that major section of your brain, but what we are going to explore in greater detail here is your limbic system, which sits just below your cerebrum. This is the part of your brain that is connected to emotions and memories.

Your limbic brain includes the olfactory bulb, amygdala and hippocampus.

How You Smell: The Olfactory Bulb

The olfactory bulb is part of your limbic system, and connects smell and memories. It is this system that forms your sense of smell within your brain. Advanced age, viral infections, exposure to toxic chemicals, head trauma and neurodegenerative diseases can all be a cause of disruption to it. This system has multiple purposes, which include using smell to detect toxic hazards, pheromones and food. Smell occurs when the source of the scent binds to specific olfactory receptor sites located within your nose.

In research done at Brown University, it was found that there was the greatest activation in the amygdala and hippocampus, suggesting that smell triggers strong emotions and memories, as well as triggers brain activity strongly linked to both.[40] While this study only had five participants, it does suggest the importance of being able to smell, and the possibility of using this system positively to support better emotions and memories, and deeper sleep.

How You Handle Stress Is Linked to Your Brain

Your amygdala is also a part of your limbic system, which connects your higher and lower brain functions. It influences your behaviour and is deeply associated with your emotional reactions to any situation, especially when you react with fear, anger or anxiety. There is a lot of research on emotions, and how they differ between the amygdala and the prefrontal cortex. The activation of the amygdala can influence impulsive decisions,[41] while the prefrontal cortex can make your decisions more deliberate and goal-directed.[42] One study found that self-regulation, being able to take conscious decisions, and goal directions are crucial for consequential outcomes in physical and mental health.[43]

You might have been exposed to various situations through your life which were disturbing. Developmental memories are crucial to how your amygdala behaves, and might explain why you react with heightened panic to particular situations. Poor sleep can be caused by the inability to neutralize emotional distress.

Here's what I want you to take away from this:

1. When you sleep, you should be able to neutralize memories, painful emotions and trauma.
2. Sleep is deeply connected to how you remember your experiences and might also be essential to getting over traumatic emotional episodes. Restless sleep prevents that alchemy of neutralizing bad emotions. In turn, traumatic emotions cause poor sleep.

3. The olfactory bulb is also part of the limbic brain, and therefore, there is a strong connection between smell, emotions and sleep. We will look at this later in the chapter on aromatherapy.

The Function of the Hippocampus

Your hippocampus is also part of your limbic system and is the neural pathway for transforming any experience into a memory. While memory is logically your brain's ability to encode, store and retrieve experiences, memories can also be real, imagined, dreamt or embellished.

Memories can be sensory, short-term and long-term. Sleep is crucial to convert short-term emotional experiences to long-term memories in the hippocampus.[44]

Memories are especially established in deep sleep.[45] During the REM of sleep, you dream. At this time, the part of your brain which is most active is your limbic brain!

The Potent Power of Aromatherapy

Smell influences your limbic brain. You can use smell to choose your emotions, influence and modulate how you react to stress or fear, and thus subconsciously impact your behaviour the next day!

1. Essential oils are an ancient wonder and have been used for thousands of years. The National Association for Holistic Aromatherapy (NAHA) defines aromatherapy as 'the therapeutic application or the medicinal use of aromatic substance for holistic health'.
2. Aromatherapy from the perspective of Ayurveda is a tool to balance the three doshas. They work like herbs. If we look at

the qualities of vata, pitta and kapha, and use the principle of opposites bring balance, we can find the right blend. Work with a practitioner to find what this is for you.

3. When smell reaches your brain, it influences your limbic system. The smell then influences your emotions, heart rate, blood pressure, memories, emotions, stress and hormone balance.
4. Aromatherapy was born from the connection between smell and the brain. When you use essential oils, they directly travel via the olfactory channel to your brain, and different oils create different emotions, once again showing the connection between the limbic brain to emotions and feelings. They are also deeply linked to memories. You probably remember the aroma of a particular incense that your grandmother used at home that made you feel calm and safe.
5. Ancient Greeks used lavender in their baths for its relaxing and soothing properties. Remember the story of Hypnos? One story goes he was surrounded by sleep-inducing opiates. Think of using lavender in a bath, where soaking in water can soothe your nervous system and reduce inflammation.
6. There are so many aroma oils associated with better sleep, including lavender, ylang-ylang, vetiver, frankincense and bergamot. I suggest reading books by Dr Eric Zielinski, who has written the section below.
7. You might find that you connect to one specific essential oil more than another.
8. There are several ways to use essential oils. When I have calls, I inhale their scent and try to intentionally breathe in the calmness they offer. I also just scatter a few drops on my table. You can use a diffusor or sprinkle a few drops diluted with water on your pillow.

Drifting into Dreamland: The Power of Essential Oils to Induce Restful Sleep

It's recommended to get between seven to nine hours of sleep each night. However, if you're like most people, you'll spend a good portion of your night tossing and turning, struggling to get to sleep.

One option for a better night's sleep is aromatherapy. Aromatherapy is easy to perform as part of a night-time ritual—it's often as simple as massaging essential oils on to your skin or using a diffuser. It could be exactly what you need to induce relaxation and enjoy the restful slumber that comes with it.

Aromatherapy Aids Sleep

Aromatherapy is a powerful holistic practice with several documented benefits. Practised right, it can help alleviate stress, manage pain, improve digestion, fight bacteria and much more. One of the better-studied benefits of aromatherapy is its ability to induce restful sleep. Essential oils have been clinically shown to help relax a person's body and calm their mind, allowing key circadian processes to take over.

The result is a body that *wants* to rest and is *ready* to rest. One 2010 study[46] even found that the scent of jasmine may be more effective than synthetic sleep aids when it comes to inducing sleep, showing how powerful our natural physiological response to aromatherapy can be. Using essential oils encourages us to shed our stress, and our weary bodies reap the benefits as we unclench and rest easy.

Inducing Relaxation through Aromatherapy

Aromatherapy is a practice so simple anyone can do it, and there are several ways to experiment with the soothing power of essential oils.

One popular method involves putting a few drops of an essential oil, like lavender or Roman chamomile, into a water diffuser and letting it run at night before you go to bed to unwind or while you sleep to promote proper rest. Diffusers effectively disperse the essential oil into a mist that permeates throughout your room. When you inhale the vapours, a cascade of wonderful events occur as your sense of smell (olfactory system) stimulates the brain to promote peace and calm.

However, diffusers aren't the only option when using essential oils to induce sleep.

Using essential oils topically has a similar effect in that you will inhale the oils as they are applied on your skin and, because they are transdermal, they will be absorbed into your bloodstream. Try mixing three drops of clary sage or geranium essential oil with one teaspoon of a carrier like coconut oil and give yourself a gentle neck rub or foot massage. Or, better yet, have someone massage you while you rest and decompress from a long, stressful day!

The Best Essential Oils for Sleep

While everyone has a different preference when it comes to essential oils, there are several that work well for inducing a good night's rest. Some of the most common include:

- **Lavender** is well-known for its stress reduction benefits.
- **Roman chamomile** has been used since ancient times to help reduce anxiety.
- **Bergamot** can reduce anxiety and boost mood.
- **Valerian** is often used as a treatment for insomnia.
- **Clary sage** and **geranium** are popular oils for women's health and stress management.

Get to Sleep, Stay Asleep, Wake Up Refreshed

Don't spend another night tossing and turning in bed. Unmanaged stress and anxiety are usually the culprits behind poor sleep, and essential oils can not only help manage the symptoms of insomnia, but these root causes as well!

Dr Eric Zielinski, D.C.
Author, *The Essential Oils Apothecary: Advanced Strategies and Protocols for Chronic Disease and Conditions*

Healing Routine to Improve Your Sense of Smell and Support Sleep

Even if you've had major problems with your sleep, be reassured that it is possible to restore deep sleep rhythms using your sense of smell.

1. Make sure that you have enough good probiotics. To support your brain health, you need to support your gut health.[47] Consuming probiotics can result in measurable change in

brain activity. Ayurveda has a spiced buttermilk called takra. It is believed that buttermilk is closest in essence to the human gut composition.

2. See that you are never deficient in omega-3 fatty acids. You require omega-3 to send blood to your brain and improve circulation in your brain. It also plays a key role in the quality of sleep via several mechanisms.[48]
3. Your brain is made up of 70 per cent fat and it requires healthy fats to stay healthy. Your body needs healthy fats even to keep cholesterol at healthy levels. Ghee is fantastic for all doshas. Kapha body constitutions may need less fats. Focus on keeping digestion robust. This is the key.
4. Spice it up! Spices are potent brain healers. They decrease brain inflammation and improve blood flow to your brain, preventing congestion in your nasal and glymphatic systems. Spices are also the way to support kapha dosha.
5. Exercise well! Exercise increases BDNF, or brain-derived neurotrophic factor, which is like a growth hormone for your brain. In fact, your body produces growth hormones when you sleep. I speak about this in detail in the section on locomotion. This is one more link to kapha dosha.
6. Practise jal neti and nasyam each morning, and anuloma viloma at some point during the day.

13

Therapies for Your Sense of Smell

Do you take a few moments every night to smell the clean sheets and the essential oil, and breathe in the calmness of these scents? What essential oils speak to your soul? Think of the benefits of each oil, and see which one merges with the intention that you have for yourself and your soul. What fragrant oils evoke memories for you?

There is so much you can do. Here are some great ways to support your sense of smell.

Replenish Micronutrients

Brain health is critical to everything. My advice would be to follow the main protocol I have laid out at the end of this book, include whatever supports balanced vata and kapha dosha, and only then look at replenishing micronutrients for reducing sinus, for the health of your glymphatic system and limbic brain health. Vata influences kapha and pitta dosha. It is wise to make vata your friend.

GABA

GABA, or γ-Aminobutyric acid, is the main inhibitory neurotransmitter in the brain. Research strongly suggests it is important for reducing stress and enhancing sleep. I suggest working with a health practitioner for this.

Sadhana or Therapies

If you feel that your sense of smell requires a sadhana or daily effort, then add the following practice into your daily life:

Jal Neti

Jal neti is the process of cleansing your nasal passage with salt water. It has been a part of yoga since time immemorial.

How to:

1. Use a copper neti or stainless steel pot. Make sure the water you use is lukewarm and as salty as your tears. Salt is crucial, as salt water is not easily absorbed via delicate blood vessels.
2. Tilt your head to a side and gently pour the water through one nostril so it comes out of the other. Making a sound helps you close off the throat.
3. Repeat this with the other nostril. It is important to not inhale the water as you pour it in.
4. Once you are done, always hang your head for a few moments and gently blow out the excess water through each nostril, until you feel clear. It is ideal to follow with one drop of nasyam oil in each nostril.

Please consult a trained practitioner for further advice. Jal neti can help brain health as regular cleansing improves the efficiency of breathing, supports reduction in inflammation within the sinus,[49] adenoids and mucous membranes, keeps the olfactory nerve healthy, soothes nerves within the olfactory bulb and has a soothing effect on your brain.

Breathing and Pranayama

Your brain requires oxygen. Only water, carbon dioxide and oxygen are allowed to pass through the tightly knit epithelial cells of your blood brain barrier, which is a microscopic barrier that keeps your nervous system safe. If your brain does not receive adequate amounts of oxygen, then brain function will diminish.

When your nose is constantly stuffy and you are unable to breathe properly, chances are high that you will be breathing more from your mouth, which is very harmful.

Breath work is another wonderful, ancient tool that supports glymphatic flow and brain health. Of course, breath has been an important topic of discussion, but here I'm going to speak about one specific type of breath, which is the anuloma viloma, or the alternate nostril breath. Look at it as three parts: Your inhalation, retained breath and exhalation.

How to practice the anuloma viloma:

1. Fold the first two fingers of your right hand and use your thumb to close the right nostril and the ring finger to close your left nostril.
2. When you first begin, breathe in through your left nostril for four counts and hold your breath for a count of eight.

3. Then exhale through your right nostril, counting to eight.
4. Inhale through your right nostril for four counts, hold your breath for eight and then exhale through your left nostril for another eight. This is one round.

For more advanced practices, consult a trained practitioner. Anuloma viloma is an excellent practice to slow down your breath and move into a more parasympathetic nervous system function, where you can rest, digest and heal.

Nasyam

Ayurveda has some wonderful ancient tools for glymphatic clearing. Nasyam is a medicated oil which is dropped into each nostril while your head is hanging upside down. When you breathe in the medicated oil, it starts to instantly clear glymphatic congestion via your nostrils. Sometimes, you even end up sneezing powerfully! Follow jal neti with one drop of nasyam. If you have high blood pressure and cannot hang the head back, take a few drops on your finger and gently wipe the inside of each nostril with it after neti.

Pratyahara to Rest Your Sense of Smell

Adding practices of breath restraint into your breath work or pranayama can be a way to withdraw and rest your sense of smell. If you add restraining your breath to your practice, the rate of gaseous exchange in your lungs is greatly increased. What this means is that more oxygen from your lungs will go into your bloodstream and more carbon dioxide from the blood is passed into your lungs for elimination. It might take some time to be able to do this comfortably if you have challenges with sinus and the glymph. First, work on restoring this system and then add this to your practice. If you have high blood pressure, you will need to avoid all breath retention.

> ### Colourful Foods and Lifestyle Habits for Brain Health
>
> Can you make your mind even sharper than it is if it is at maximum capacity? Probably not. But can you buffer your brain against mild decline and even more severe reduced function due to dementia by making some changes in what you eat and how you live? Research would say a resounding *yes*!
>
> Here are some tips to boost your brain health.
>
> **Eat blue and purple whole foods**, such as blackberries, blueberries, plums, purple potatoes and more. Look for purple varieties of your favourite fruits and vegetables, such as purple cauliflower, cabbage, carrots, kale and grapes. Blue and purple plant foods are rich in antioxidants, in particular those that protect the brain and nervous system from oxidative stress and inflammation caused by free radical damage. Anthocyanins, blue–purple pigments found in plant foods, are antioxidant flavonoids that can cross the blood brain barrier to exert their benefits on brain cells, including improving vascular function, blood flow and cognitive function.
>
> **Spice up your food!** Turmeric, which contains curcumin, is a powerful anti-inflammatory and antioxidant

compound. Researchers have theorized that the historically low rates of dementia in India is because of our use of turmeric. When it comes to the brain, not only can curcumin protect the brain cells, but it can also prevent the build-up of the protein beta-amyloid, one of the hallmarks of dementia.

Eat like you live in the Mediterranean. Studies have shown that the more one can follow a Mediterranean way of eating (i.e., fish, fresh fruits and vegetables, nuts, legumes, spices, extra virgin olive oil), the more our brains may be protected from decline and dementia, especially if we have Type 2 diabetes, where the risk increases twofold. Since brain decline is linked to blood sugar balance, it's important to consider a 'modified' Mediterranean diet, so you do not eat much of the high glycaemic impact carbohydrates that can spike blood sugar. Put the focus on high-fibre legumes, non-gluten whole grains and nuts for sugar-stabilizing action.

Let go of stress. Stress shrinks certain parts of the brain. Therefore, it's essential to choose a stress-modulation practice that you enjoy, whether it is yoga, meditation or mindfulness. Studies show that yoga may have some role in promoting a healthy mood and meditation sessions can do the same. In fact, one study showed that the more one meditates, the better one's mood and the lower the amount of inflammation in the body—two thumbs up for the brain! Meditation can also help with promoting healthy blood flow to the brain, which means you're delivering more oxygen and nutrients to the precious tissue. Mindfulness practice assists in fine-tuning one's ability to pay attention and even

> leads to increases in brain grey matter density, which is a good thing if your brain is stressed and shrunk.
>
> Keeping your grey matter bright with brilliance is definitely within reach, no matter what your age! These simple lifestyle steps will shine light on your path forward into the decades to come.[50 51 52 53 54 55 56]
>
> —Deanna Minich, PhD, nutritionist, educator, and author of *Whole Detox*

How Tara Improved Sleep Using Her Sense of Smell

Tara started to calm kapha dosha by avoiding heavy foods, like cheese, at night. She takes five minutes each morning after brushing her teeth to practice jal neti and follows it with a drop of nasyam. She makes sure that she walks every day to keep kapha moving. Each evening before dinner, she spends ten minutes practising some alternate nostril breathing. At night, she applies the principles of aromatherapy to her bedroom, which helps her feel calm. She is amazed at how improving the health of her nose changed her pattern of breathing. The shift from mouth breathing to nose breathing has been game-changing for her!

PART 5

The Fourth Sense: Touch

14

Touch, Connection and Oxytocin

Reverend Kelly Isola talks about the symbolism of touch in the most profound way. She says, 'But the deep, exquisite risk is to humbly lift the veil draped so long ago that we fearfully kept ourselves wrapped up in, and let life touch us, refresh us, renew us, and rearrange us.'[57]

How is touch linked to poor sleep? Oxytocin supports sleep recovery and deep healing. The bidirectional relationship between cortisol and oxytocin is relevant and inspiring.

What Is Oxytocin?

Oxytocin is a hormone that is normally produced in your hypothalamus and released by your posterior pituitary gland. It plays an immense role in social bonding, sexual reproduction and childbirth. Have you thought about what it means physiologically to fall in love? Some fascinating research describes it as a release of adrenaline, dopamine, oxytocin and serotonin![58]

How Is Touch Linked to Poor Sleep?

Myra had urticaria, which are bright red inflamed patches on the skin, all over her body. Her eyes would swell shut during the worst of it. Her lips would swell as well. On some parts of her body, there were red welts that would burn badly, and her entire body would feel immense pain. In her twenties, Myra struggled also with the emotional pain of feeling she wasn't normal.

The first episode went on for many years, beginning when she was just nine and lasting until she was almost twenty. After that, Myra seemed to have had a brief year or two of relief before it was severely triggered again. This lasted for another few years. It seemed to come in waves, lasting for a few years and then staying dormant for a short while before flaring up again.

> **Sleep and Skin**
>
> Any negative reactions in relationships, especially in women, is linked to increased cortisol.[59] Any good form of touch increases oxytocin and promotes healing.[60] Stress can be physical, with symptoms like skin flare-ups; it can be nutritional stress due to deficiencies; it can be emotional stress, or immune stress from allergies and candida, or stress from trauma.

Understanding the Skin and Your Sense of Touch

If you've suffered from any condition like urticaria, eczema, psoriasis, acne or candida overgrowth, this entire chapter will resonate with you deeply. Maybe it's not severe, and your skin just feels itchy all the time or is sensitive to new creams, changes in the environment or stress. Yet, you cannot ignore this for the rest of your life. Do you find yourself waking up with severe itching or pain on your skin? Do the symptoms bother you so much that you cannot get through life without an antihistamine?

What Happens with Skin Inflammation?

There are several factors which connect skin challenges to poor sleep. Here are some of those connections.

Skin inflammation can be triggered by nutrient deficiencies, gut permeability, liver congestion, vata aggravation, pitta aggravation, food allergens when digestion is weak, exposure to toxins, synthetic clothes, itching, sweating, excessive heat, excessive cold, adrenal issues, hormonal imbalance, a feeling of isolation, pathogenic bacteria, poor microbiome, poor sleep, histamine elevation and stress.

Symptoms may worsen at night, affecting your sleep or making whatever sleep you get poor in quality. Why should this be so? The circadian rhythm regulates hormones and chemicals in your body. The rhythm itself can cause more blood flow to your skin at night, increasing skin temperature and making you feel extremely uncomfortable, thereby increasing the level of cytokines, which are immune response cells. This increases inflammation at night, lowering levels of corticosteroid, which help lower inflammation, and making the skin drier and more susceptible to symptoms.[61] Pitta time is 10.00 p.m. to 2.00 a.m. and this can aggravate the issue further, especially in situations of imbalance.

This situation can become worse in perimenopause, as low levels of oestrogen can cause dry skin, worsening other symptoms. Perimenopause is at the vata time of life, and vata aggravation is common too. This also explains the sleep issues that occur at that time. When you have skin issues like eczema, it is common to have severe flare-ups at night, impacting as many as 85 per cent of people with inflammatory conditions.[62] In sleep, however poor, it's also possible that you scratch yourself, causing more irritation and even bleeding.

Can Anger Be Linked to Skin Health?

Emotions play a major role in skin health. Specific systems can be linked to specific emotions. Anger has been linked to liver health in both Ayurveda and traditional Chinese medicine.[63] Symptoms of pitta aggravation include skin inflammation and anger as well!

Those with constant angry outbursts have been found to have elevated inflammatory markers[64] or are physiologically in a state of inflammation. Ayurveda understood this connection long ago.

A deficiency in omega-3 fatty acids can put a strain on your brain and lead to brain inflammation.[65] Omega-3 is required for getting blood supply to the brain, and for production and transmission of your neurotransmitters.

I know how frustrating chronic skin inflammation can be! When we learn more about cortisol and oxytocin in this section, you'll be able to understand your sense of touch through the lens of histamine and pitta. That understanding will help you use your sense of touch in powerful ways to support your sleep.

When you care for your skin, whether you have challenges with your skin or not, you deeply support an increase in oxytocin and a decrease in cortisol. It also calms down vata dosha and pitta dosha, helping sleep.

A Healing Routine to Overcome Skin Inflammation

Here, I break down some specific steps for your skin recovery before we go into the section on using touch positively.

1. Temporarily eliminate foods such as tomatoes, cheese, chocolate, wine, beer, fermented foods, soy sauce, bone broth, aged meat, avocado, coffee, tea, eggplant, pineapple, strawberry, litchi, mango, yeast, mushroom, mustard and dried fruit for a period of two to three months. All these foods are triggers of skin inflammation as they are high in histamines.[66] Many of the high-histamine foods overlap with pitta-aggravating foods. Pitta-aggravating foods are those which are hot, spicy, sour and acidic, fermented foods, caffeine and alcohol.
2. Restore the circadian rhythm. Skin health thrives on a sense of routine, so sticking to a more predictable schedule can help to keep your mind and body both cool and grounded.
3. Aim for the right form of and time to exercise. When the skin is inflamed, it is common to feel your symptoms getting worse after heavy exercise, especially if you are in the sun or getting internally hot. This is also a pitta-aggravating aspect. Exercise when it is cooler, like early in the morning. Activities such as yoga, swimming, walking and tai chi will support a healing journey.
4. Meditate. Try a zen Buddhist moving meditation, where you feel the ground beneath your feet on a long walk and coordinate your footsteps with your breath.
5. Shield yourself from the heat. Try and find ways to stay cool. Don't be out in bright sunlight. Wear cooling fabrics that touch your skin and are soothing. Avoid synthetic clothes. Wearing loose and lightweight clothes will help as well.
6. Enjoy a cool bath. Soak in a tub of cool water with some tea and essential oils added to it. Try adding jasmine oil. Remember to wear cooling colours like whites, blues and soothing greens. Excess sun spikes histamine and imbalances pitta.

7. Soothe your skin. Try aloe gel as it has long been used for its capability to rejuvenate the skin while being cooling. If your skin does not flare up, the best support for it is abhyanga several times per week.
8. Drink half a glass of aloe juice on an empty stomach. Consuming a teaspoon of aloe also calms pitta dosha.
9. Keep your bedroom cool. Sweating or feeling hot will not help soothe skin inflammation nor will it promote sleep.

> The link between symptoms of skin inflammation and poor sleep is histamine.[67] It is a compound released by your mast cells, which are white blood cells. If you have histamine intolerance due to the inability to break them down, then histamine elevation can trigger skin issues and spoil sleep. If you lack DAO, an enzyme required to break down histamines, or have some genetic liver challenges, it can result in the inability to metabolize and excrete histamine. The Ayurvedic perspective of pitta imbalance overlaps in some ways with histamine elevation.
>
> Mast cells play a key role in circadian rhythms.[68] There are histamine receptors in the brain which affect serotonin, dopamine and GABA. When you have a histamine elevation and you are histamine intolerant, you can experience anxiety, skin inflammation and poor sleep. Histamine can reach its peak in the middle of the night or early in the morning. Therefore, your skin condition can provide a clue about potential histamine intolerance and can point towards why the quality of your sleep is so poor. Lowering histamine can then be the path forward towards correcting your specific sleep challenges.

15

The Seesaw of Oxytocin and Cortisol

Touch is an intimate sense, more than any other, and is a metaphor for connection. Touching someone you love, when you hug them or hold their hand, releases oxytocin, which leaves you feeling tranquil and reduces cortisol elevation to promote good sleep.

Symbolically, you can also be touched by emotion, and when you feel emotions that support peace and rest, it supports your sleep. Touch is also connected to healthy hormones. Oxytocin supports healthy hormones. If you have faced the opposite as aggression, it can elevate cortisol and keep you in a permanent state of fight or flight.

When stress throws off your immune system, your body responds in certain situations by sending out histamine to keep away the problem at hand, which is stress.

The sensitive connection between stress and skin conditions have been well documented since ancient times. It is the first barrier in your immune system, and as such is responsible for maintaining the balance between the external environment and internal tissue. Your skin participates in the stress response using what is called a local HPA axis, nerve endings, mast cells and immune cells. There is constant feedback and crosstalk between your brain and your skin. Till today, there is no proven medical treatment that can prevent or treat stress-induced skin inflammation. Skin mast cells in turn produce stress hormones, leading to a stress-induced inflammatory cycle.[69]

Can Aggression Impact Your Physiology?

When you hear the phrase 'bad touch', you tend to think of what you tell children, on how to stay away from a stranger touching them. Bad touch can also be aggression and abuse.

Myra started to experience severe skin inflammation once more within a few years of getting married and, no matter what she tried, she could not get herself into that ideal state of remission. The one thing that she could not change was her level of stress.

Any threatening behaviour or aggression repeatedly directed towards you is correlated with having psychological difficulties, activation of the HPA axis, loss of function in your hippocampus, increased cortisol levels and alterations in the HPA axis. Studies are trying to find the link between aggression and cortisol.[70]

Cortisol levels typically rise upon waking and start to decline progressively through the day. In the journal *Psychoneuroendocrinology*, researchers found disrupted cortisol rhythm to be at a slower decline in the afternoon and at higher than normal levels later. It was discovered that aggressive touch had an adverse impact on HPA function and resulted in poor resilience to stress.[71] There was also a thought that those with dysfunctional cortisol and elevated stress had a greater tendency towards any kind of interpersonal violence.

You might not have faced anything as severe as aggression or violence, as in the studies mentioned above, but any form of aggressive touch can lead to a similar elevation of cortisol, and the inability to manage and tame skin inflammation.

Soothing Touch and Oxytocin Secretion

I'll share another story before I take you through research on the impact of good touch on skin health and sleep. At the time Myra met her current husband and became good friends with him, she had forgotten what it was like to feel a sense of safety. By safety, I mean a feeling of being safe emotionally, physically and even financially.

In the section on sound, I explained how sound can be memories and how Tamara would wake up when she heard the cupboard door open. The reason this happens is the HPA programming after years of immense stress. At that moment, a loving hug can calm you down, and the oxytocin release can lower cortisol and help you go back to sleep.

What is this magical hormone called oxytocin and what does it do? How is it so powerful to healing?

Touch, which is healing and gentle, raises oxytocin and that creates immense positive physiological change. Many things play a role in oxytocin release. When parents hug more and bond more through pregnancy, the mother can heal from childbirth much faster. It is oxytocin that makes a mother bond with her new baby. In fact, lower oxytocin might be correlated with increased risk of postnatal depression, and as such research is attempting to find a connection between the use of oxytocin in prevention or treatment of postpartum depression.[72]

Before you are born, it is your mother who flushes you with oxytocin and protects your gut. The release of oxytocin can combat stress and induce anti-stress effects such as lowered blood pressure and cortisol levels. In turn, it improves positive social interaction and promotes healing.[73]

Oxytocin protects your gut, helps your liver, signals lactation, helps treat physical and emotional pain and helps you bond. It also supports your vagus nerve, which I talk about later.

The most important takeaway from this section is that aggressive touch can spike cortisol, but gentle and loving touch can increase oxytocin and lower cortisol, which in turn reduces overall inflammation. There are various ways of using your sense of touch to increase oxytocin and restore sleep.

When you feel the warmth of the water as you bathe or the hug of a loved one, your brain floods your body with oxytocin, which can lull you into sleep.

Oxytocin can be released by hugging, bonding, orgasms, massage, meditation, feeling cold water on your face and any form of gentle touch. Isn't that a powerful way to use touch for healing, recovery and better sleep?

What Is the Right Temperature for Sleep?

In a sleeping space, suggestions for temperature generally range between 16–21 degrees Celsius. However, I disagree. We are all unique. Excess cold when someone has vata aggravation can be worse. Begin where it is comfortable for you, but cooler is better.

Your hypothalamus regulates your core body temperature according to the circadian rhythm. It ranges between 36–38 degrees Celsius during a twenty-four-hour cycle. Sleep begins when your core body temperature drops. A warmer core body temperature is associated with feeling more active.

Having an oil massage with the right oil and the temperature of bath water can better regulate your body temperature. I talk more about this in the section on abhyanga at the end of this chapter.

An Evening Routine to Raise Oxytocin and Improve Sleep

If you combine this specific evening routine with the protocols to lower skin inflammation, you will find promising ways to restore your sleep and promote deep inner healing.

1. Massage therapy has multiple positive effects on your biochemistry, including lowered cortisol and skin inflammation, increased serotonin, dopamine and increased oxytocin.[74] Studies have found that after a massage, oxytocin increased dramatically, while stress hormones decreased rapidly.[75]
2. Have a bath before your dinner. It is even better if you have a massage beforehand.
3. Spend some time hugging someone you love. It could be your baby, your partner or a dear friend. If you have a partner, spending some time just hugging and touching can be very helpful for sleep. Dedicate time towards this. The mother and child bond is probably the most profound to oxytocin. When I hug my son, peace descends into my body and mind, and I am left feeling a sense of emotional stillness.
4. How can I miss sexual gratification? Orgasms raise oxytocin levels and support good sleep.[76]
5. Meditation can also increase oxytocin.[77] I have several guided meditations on my podcast, which you can easily do while sitting on your bed.

Creating Your Zen Zone to Soothe Your Sense of Touch

To use the sense of touch to promote sleep, look towards creating a sacred sleep sanctuary:

1. When choosing your sheets, try different fabrics to see what appeals to you. The sense of touch is powerful.
2. Your rug is the last thing that you step on before you get to bed at night and the first thing you step on when you wake up. So, take time to choose one which feels comforting and promotes a safe space.
3. Take time to choose razais, and here is where I would really encourage you to go with natural fabrics, like organic cotton and linen, as it allows your skin to breathe.
4. Another thing to consider is temperature. Regular abhyanga with the right oil allows you to better regulate your own body temperature.
5. Finally, your mattress is a very big deal! Too many people are ignoring this and using a mattress that may be a decade old or more. Most stores allow you to lie down and try out mattresses, and it is crucial to invest time and money in this as it is going to be the primary source of touch to support sleep. Make sure to also rotate your mattress every couple of weeks, bringing the head to the foot and the foot to the head, to encourage even wearing down. Mattresses are sprayed with flame retardants to pass a test where they must last a minute under an open flame. This is a major toxin. The coils in mattresses are like metal detectors that will amplify any electromagnetic field (EMF) radiation that is around. EMF impacts your pineal gland and your circadian rhythm. Sunning your mattress can be very helpful.
6. If you have a loving partner, enjoy a loving embrace that produces oxytocin.

Do you take time to experience touch in your sleep sanctuary? Does the comfort of your bed evoke any memories? Do you feel comforted in your bed? Do you take time to feel its texture? Do you notice the softness of your pillow and how it feels soothing at the end of a long, tiring day? As you take a deep breath, do you feel your breath moving through your body and soothing you deep within?

16

Therapies for Your Sense of Touch

Your skin is the largest organ in your body and keeping it healthy is much more than mere aesthetics. If it's physiological skin inflammation and skin conditions that prevent sleep, then turn to supplements for those.

Replenish Micronutrients for Skin and Oxytocin

Also remember that supplements are not everything. They are meant only to support nutrition and practices to lower stress, and those that use touch help increase oxytocin, lower cortisol and improve sleep. I always suggest working with the foundational aspects of food, lifestyle, exercise, abhyanga and relaxation before looking at supplements.

Valerian Root

Valerian root has been used extensively for better sleep. It can be taken in the evening or a few hours before bedtime. It can suppress physical and psychological stress responses by modulating the hippocampus and amygdala.[78]

Quercetin

If your skin conditions or inflammation is caused by histamine release, quercetin can be helpful in preventing your immune cells from releasing histamine. It can be as effective, or even more, than prescription medication. It has potent antioxidant properties, fighting free radical damage. It can support immune-related skin conditions by restoring some stability to mast cells and lowering histamine release.

Sadhana or Therapies

There are beautiful practices using the sense of touch, which also bring together community, family and tribe. Some of the practices can be powerful in releasing any feelings of isolation, which can trigger immune-related skin conditions.

Having gratitude for receiving or having the knowledge of this sadhana will help you go further.

The Right Way to Do Abhyanga

Massage has been a part of many cultures. As I mentioned before, massage therapies have been found to increase oxytocin and reduce cortisol. There are amazing, ancient tools from the science of yoga and Ayurveda that are deeply supportive to health. Most of these are easily accessible, and all you need is to find the right guide. Once you learn a few ancient tools, you're equipped with skills which can help you with your health.

In India, massaging begins the day a baby is born. As part of most Indian cultures, babies are massaged every day, with different oils in different cultures, and then bathed. I recall my great-grandmother and my grandmother giving me an oil massage for as long as they were alive.

Apply a good ayurvedic oil in long, gentle movements, in a loving manner. Soft-touch massage has been associated even more than regular massages with increased oxytocin and decreased cortisol. That's proof that you really do not need a deep-tissue massage for profound effects. You need gentle applications with a soft touch. Another approach is to have a combined massage with a partner, which can improve oxytocin as well.

You can use an Ayurvedic oil like dhanwantaram tailam or chemparuthyadi tailam all over your body, and then you can use castor oil specifically over your abdominal area, the soles of your feet, the palms of your hands and on the crown of your head. This tradition is part of ancient Eastern wisdom. Warm sesame oil abhyanga is calming to vata dosha and very helpful to sleep. If it is the height of summer in a hot location, and you feel overheated, try chemparuthyadi tailam.

Lay a newspaper on the floor to avoid cleaning up afterwards. You need to apply it, soak in it and then bathe for ten minutes each.

You do not need to oil the head every day. Bathe using powdered gram flour or a gentle organic soap. You can safely do the abhyanga for your body every day if you want. Ideally, it is great in the morning, before a bath. But, if you find yourself struggling with energy during the day, keep this for early evening, before dinner.

My ancient abhyanga masterclass and blissful sleep programme have detailed recommendations for oils based on body constitution, season and location, recipes for bath powder based on constitution and more detailed information on using abhyanga for the right movement of energy.

Cool Bath

Cool water not only combats skin inflammation, but also increases oxytocin, calms pitta, quells histamine spikes and lowers cortisol.

If you do not have access to a bathtub, then fill a bucket with cool water, boiled tea leaves or rose petals, Epsom salt and rose oil. Imagine the cool water releasing all your stress. Try to feel a blue light radiating from the cool water and cutting the fire on any inflamed patches on your body. We are all unique. This can be helpful in the summer, or for someone with excess pitta or histamine spikes. It might imbalance someone with excess vata or kapha, especially in winter. Remember the principles of like increases like and opposites bring balance. Try this just once if you struggle with symptoms of skin inflammation or rashes.

Stroking Your Pet

My dearest Dalmatian, Moksha, was just five years old and passed away shortly before this book went into publication. When he was three years old, he was bitten by something, and could not walk properly and kept falling. The doctor said that he had a neurological deficit in three legs, and an MRI revealed myelitis, or inflammation in his spine. He started falling for no reason at all and crumpled into a heap. He became depressed and his eyes lacked the mischievous light that was ever-present before.

Eventually, he became a quadriplegic. One afternoon, I was feeling stressed and tired. He was looking depressed. I crawled under my dining table, lay down with my body close to his back and stroked his face for half an hour. I felt blissful and relaxed after that. He fell into a calm sleep, and woke up and licked my face. If you have dogs or cats, or any animal you love, I don't need to tell you how powerful stroking them might be. I'm sure you don't need any reminder to do this as well.

Weighted Blankets

It is so strange that weighted blankets have become so popular in the sleep world today. Decades ago in India, the practice of filling cotton blankets until they were as big as mini mattresses was very common. Weighted blankets have been found to improve sleep quality through altered tactile inputs.[79] It all comes back to calming vata dosha. Think of swaddling a baby and how the baby sleeps with a feeling of being held.

What happens is that the extra weight is very similar to therapeutic techniques like massage. It helps you feel calmer, prompting a parasympathetic shift. It can also be a helpful tool for someone who does not have a loved one at home and feels isolated. However, if someone struggles with moving this heavy weight, then caution must be used. This includes very small children, someone struggling with sudden movements, those with more complex sleep challenges such as sleep apnoea or those who are claustrophobic.

Sense Withdrawal to Soothe Touch

Asanas, as you know, are postures that remain comfortable and steady. There are many postures, and I see many people struggling to master a complex one. Yet, yoga postures never existed for someone to perfect all of them. In fact, it is said that no one can achieve mastery over all of them in a lifetime. There is a belief among older yoga practitioners that the reason so many asanas exist is to loosen all parts of your body, so that you can sit still for meditation for longer periods of time. Isn't that beautiful? It takes away all the goals associated with postures in yoga.

The best way to restrain your sense of touch for some time and give it rest is to sit still in a steady posture, one as simple as sitting cross-legged. Staying still and steady in that pose can rest your sense of touch, allowing you to perceive and analyse it in a more sensitive way afterwards.

How Myra Improved Her Sleep Using the Sense of Touch

Myra started to calm excess pitta dosha and histamine spikes by reducing fiery, fermented and pungent foods. She drinks a quarter cup of aloe juice thrice a day to help her body calm down. She makes sure that she exercises early in the morning, before the sun comes up. She is intentional about her abhyanga each morning. At night, she gives herself space to relax and feel the softness of her cool cotton sheets. Over time, her skin calmed down, her anger reduced and her sleep improved.

PART 6

The Fifth Sense: Taste

17

Taste, Gratitude and Fasting

The health of your tongue, mouth, vagus nerve and oral cavity are critical to good sleep. While you might not have a specific digestive concern or any condition, remember that the gut is central to every system, and is a key player in determining the quality of sleep you get. The food you eat is also crucial for your overall health.

What Did Watching *The Parent Trap* **Teach Me?**

Have you watched the movie *The Parent Trap*? Identical twins Hallie and Annie are separated after their parents' divorce. Years later, they run into each other at a summer camp. After fighting with each other and being sentenced to isolation until camp is over, they discover that they are twin sisters who cannot naturally hate each other, as much as they try. They switch places and live each other's lives with the opposite parent. Finally, they bring the parents back together, for Hallie and Annie belong together. They discovered quickly that they are identical, that what upsets one upsets the other and that they want the best for each other, no matter what.

Your gut and your brain are like Hallie and Annie, separated at some point but identical, and what upsets one upsets the other. What supports one benefits the other as well! In early embryonic stages, the same clump of tissue is the root of your gut and your brain. As the embryo evolves and grows, the brain goes towards the crown and the gut moves to the centre. This doesn't mean that they are not connected after that. Your brain and your gut are connected via the vagus nerve, which is called the wanderer, as it moves through your body, reaching many areas, controlling a great deal in the process.

Vagus is the nerve that carries information from your brain to your body's major systems, allowing them to decode that information, slow down, achieve a parasympathetic nervous system response and ultimately regulate themselves. It is often called the nerve of compassion. You will understand the pivotal role the vagus nerve plays in regulating your sleep. Modulating the vagus nerve with practices like meditation have therapeutic, calming and anti-inflammatory effects.[80]

How Is Taste Linked to Poor Sleep?

Rahul slept poorly and always had a bitter taste in his mouth that prevented him from enjoying food, he found undigested food in his stool and had digestive distress that ranged between acidity and indigestion. He was frustrated because he had tried everything from eating small meals frequently to playing around with his diet. He struggled to fall asleep and then he awoke frequently with high anxiety.

He used to eat very slowly as a child, until his mother started to lose patience with him for making her wait so long before she could clear up. One day, she lost her temper at him and threw his plate on the floor. Ever since, he started gobbling up his food. He became more anxious and that ruined his sleep.

Understanding Taste

Digestion begins when you smell food and it sends a signal to the brain via the olfactory channel to begin secreting saliva with digestive enzymes within the mouth before you even taste food.

Taste is not just about satisfying your tongue, but it also has a physiological connection to your entire digestive process. It can lead to a complex chain of reactions within your body, right from the time when you think about the wonders of food and allow your brain to begin secreting saliva in your mouth. Ayurveda talks about consuming food with all your senses, suggesting that how you digest your food is how you will digest your life. Proper digestion right from this stage is critical to good sleep.

Can a Healthy Oral Cavity Help?

The oral cavity is the first area where food meets your physiology. It consists of your cheeks, your soft and hard palates, and your tongue. Within this cavity are your salivary glands and teeth, both crucial to the digestive process. This space is the region for your sense of taste, and therefore, the health of all that is within this cavity influences taste. In Ayurveda, it is kapha dosha that is connected to the mouth.

Insulin resistance can increase upper airway collapsibility and can correlate to sleep issues.[81]

Your salivary glands are located within your oral cavity. Saliva is crucial to cleanse your mouth and teeth, and aid digestion by chemically breaking down starches and lipids while destroying any bacteria in food. Saliva secretion is stimulated by the thought, smell, sight and sound of food!

Saliva has its own pH buffering system to maintain acid–alkaline balance. It secretes bicarbonate and an enzyme called anhydrase. This enzyme not only maintains pH in your mouth, but also protects your tastebuds from premature cell death. Enzyme secretion can also be disrupted by zinc deficiency, which is extremely common. Remember Rahul suffering from a bitter taste in his mouth and being unable to taste food? That had to do with zinc deficiency.

Your teeth help you break down food, mix saliva into food, and increase the surface area of food to allow enzyme exposure, all through the practice of chewing. Ayurveda talks about how excess watery foods can put out the fire of digestion. These foods can also increase vata dosha and disrupt sleep.

The Environment of Your Mouth: The Oral Microbiome

It's very important that I go into the microbiome again in this chapter because your mouth has its own microbiome, and it plays an integral role in the health of your tongue, teeth and oral cavity.

Did you know ...

1. Some dysbiosis in the microbiome has been shown to cause many teeth infections, and there is more and more evidence to the state of the oral microbiome having a connection with many systemic diseases including cardiovascular disease, stroke and diabetes. With the understanding that these surfaces are covered by a

complex biofilm of multiple microbial communities,[82] there is more focus today on rebuilding the mouth microbiome rather than targeting a single infection, which can recur.
2. It might seem small, but the oral microbiome can impact the health of your gut and increase your chances for developing gastrointestinal conditions such as irritable bowel syndrome (IBS). It was found that people with IBS had more pathogenic bacteria, such as streptococcus, in their mouth.[83]
3. Some pathogenic bacteria in the mouth, like klebsiella, instigate inflammatory activity in the gut.[84] Those struggling with chronic liver issues were also found to have dysbiosis, most of which were found in their mouth![85]
4. Tongue diagnosis has been used as a barometer of all health in traditional Chinese medicine and Ayurveda. Some studies found that in people with chronic insomnia, the oral microbiome had significantly altered diversity and abundance.[86] It is unnecessary to analyse the tongue here. Suffice to say, having a coating on the tongue indicates suboptimal digestion and the accumulation of ama, or metabolic waste, which impacts all systems and sleep. Having cracks on the tongue can indicate dryness and increased vata.

Why Is Chewing Important?

Once you put food into your mouth and begin to taste it, you should be blown away by the immense burst of flavours that explodes in your mouth. The longer the food stays in your mouth, the better your digestion.

Chewing helps you keep food in your mouth for longer, allowing you to savour taste and easing the burden on digestion.

Lack of adequate chewing leads to weak digestion. This causes poor nutrient utilization and leads to the formation of ama, or metabolic toxins. This build-up leads to weakening of almost every system and organ, and is also a cause of all kinds of disease. *Insomnia is a symptom of ama accumulation.*

Zinc Deficiency and Sleep Connection

Zinc deficiency can impact your sleep quality. New research indicates that a deficiency of zinc, which might be reflected as poor taste, has an impact on how you sleep, how much you sleep and the overall quality of your sleep.[87]

It is unclear if zinc triggers sleep, but optimal zinc levels reduce the time it takes for you to fall asleep, increases your overall sleep time and improves sleep quality.[88] Children who have poor zinc levels in early childhood might grow into adolescents and adults with poor sleeping patterns.

Those who have poor sleep or disturbed sleep could have limited or low levels of zinc in their diet. It's also evident that sleep disorders and sleep challenges of any kind can be a result of zinc deficiency. One of the most surprising functions of zinc may be in aiding sleep regulation.[89]

18

The Vagus Nerve, Fasting and Sleep

Your vagus nerve is one of the cranial nerves that connects your brain to the rest of your body. It has two bunches of sensory nerve cell bodies and connects the brainstem to the body. Your brain houses the control centre of your nervous system and your gut is your enteric nervous system. The vagus nerve connecting the two creates the deep gut-brain axis. Your enteric nervous system is in the tissue around your oesophagus, stomach, small intestine and colon. It controls your entire gastrointestinal function. This is no small role.

The vagus nerve lets your gut feel the impact of your brain and vice versa. This can be both good and bad. This of course means that when you feel angry or depressed, you either cannot eat or your digestion is impaired, and if your digestion is impaired you feel anxious or depressed. But we forget that this also means we have great power!

Your vagus nerve plays a role in hunger, elimination, enzyme release, bronchial constriction, stimulation of peristalsis, stimulation of bile flow, intestinal blood flow and sleep. It regulates inflammatory response and supports your movement towards the parasympathetic nervous system response of your autonomic nervous system, which, as you know, is critical to how you sleep.

When you see or smell food, it stimulates a nerve impulse that sends a message to the hypothalamus. This signals to a part of your brain called the medulla oblongata, which sends out nerve impulses that travel down your vagus nerve to stimulate more saliva and gastric enzymes.

Vagal tone is key to activating this parasympathetic response. It can be measured by tracking your heart rate and breathing rate. Your heart rate speeds up a little when you breathe in and slows down when you breathe out. The greater the difference between your inhalation and your exhalation heart rates, the higher your vagal tone. This gives you tangible evidence of the impact of vagus nerve support on your sleep. A higher vagal tone means that your body can relax faster after undergoing stress. It also means that you can sleep better, so it's crucial to include practices that support vagal tone health, such as breathing with longer exhales.

Vagal Tone Support

Let us look into some easy steps for the vagus tone before we go into how to use the sense of taste positively. I want to emphasize on simple tools and practices which can be supportive in activating the parasympathetic nervous system, help with digestion, slow down the heart rate and breathing rate, and improve sleep.

1. Gratitude is great. Practising gratitude indicates to your nervous system a feeling of safety and helps condition your vagus nerve.[90]
2. Cold is thermogenesis. Cold stimulation, especially on the neck, can result in higher heart-rate variability and lower

heart rate, prompting better sleep.[91] Have caution using cold therapy as it can imbalance vata for some.
3. Deep breathing is key. If you bring in practices that support the parasympathetic response, it will improve vagal tone as well. The longer you exhale in comparison to your inhalation, the better. Count in your mind when you inhale and exhale, ensuring you breathe out for double the time you breathe in. Vagus nerve activity is modulated by respiration, and facilitated with slow exhalation and respiration cycles. Several apps on watches have breathing cues, but I find them to be too fast. In many of them, the inhalation and exhalation periods are the same.
4. Exercise. A complete yoga practice that includes inversions, forward bends, backward bends, lateral bends and twists can have a profound effect on the vagus nerve.
5. Balance your oral microbiome. Gargling not only supports your oral microbiome health, but also improves heart rate variability and vagal tone, while supporting taste.
6. Sing and hum. In the section on sound, I spoke about brahmari, which is the humming breath. That is a great practice to improve vagal tone as well.
7. Oil pulling is mentioned in detail in the chapter on therapies for your sense of taste.

Don't be overwhelmed by all of this. If you can pick one of the above and be regular with it, that itself will help you tremendously.

Can Fasting Help You Sleep?

Some years ago, I was asked to fast for an entire day by someone very dear to me.

Ancient wisdom mentions fasting as a cure for any symptom or disease in the body. By giving a much-needed rest to the digestive system, eliminating toxins from the body and cleansing it to release more energy, it was considered a way to tackle many ailments.

Sometimes, enemas were used as part of longer fasts to support detoxification. It gave the mind an opportunity to rest and slow down the entire system, allowing the body to move into a parasympathetic nervous system response. Physically, the entire system is overhauled. Mentally, you develop concentration.

The benefits of fasting are many:

1. It gives your digestive system a much-needed rest. In this manner, it also heals your gut and resets your microbiome.
2. Fasting allows for autophagy, which is a programmed cell death. Your body has the amazing capability of digesting and killing only old and worn-out cells during a fast. This allows for renewed call optimization and improved energy.
3. It raises stem cells within your bone marrow. After longer fasts, it can even replace some autoimmune cells.
4. It boosts your immune system and improves overall immune function.
5. It resets your DNA. It produces ketones which are brain healing and neuroprotective.
6. Fasting boosts growth hormone release and improves cell receptivity.
7. In the context of sleep, fasting can help reduce insulin resistance, which can support melatonin release and rise.[92]

Ancient cultures had feast and famine cycles all the time, based on drought and other natural factors. People made their body more resilient to accepting different foods, diets and times for eating.

This gave their microbiome adaptability to reset itself. When the body is forced to adapt to changes and variations in diet and taste, hormone optimization occurs.

There are many ways to introduce fasting into your life:

1. Fasting is not advised when there is vata aggravation. I have often seen people who begin with fasting struggle with sleep due to elevation of cortisol. Vata bodies are the most sensitive to fasting.
2. Fasting during seasonal change is beneficial. Short fasts are better. Longer fasts can increase dry qualities of vata. However, all body constitutions do well with concluding dinner close to sunset, which supports strong agni and balance of vata.
3. Fasting can be helpful for those with a kapha constitution. It will rest your digestive system and give your migrating motor complex time to clean. Fasting will make you really appreciate your food and enjoy subtle tastes.

If you find yourself more irritable or experiencing adrenal dysfunction, blood sugar imbalance, terrible sleep, disrupted hormones, acid reflux or anxiety, then fasting will not work for you. In this case, you can ease back for a while until you find the delicate balance that works for you. Begin with whatever you can.

How does fasting influence the quality of your sleep? Eating early in the evenings is immensely light on digestion. Once you incorporate some fasting every day, including scheduled eating, it starts to optimize the circadian rhythm. Once this is optimized, you'll find it much easier to fall asleep and stay asleep for longer.

I've found people trying to skip dinner, and all it's done is wake them up due to hunger pangs, blood sugar imbalance and cortisol spikes. It really is a delicate balance, and there should be no rush to reach an ideal state of fasting. Find whatever works for you.

I faced years of terrible sleep when I first started fasting. When I found the right methodology and incorporated the practice regularly, which was just finishing dinner before sunset, I found myself really enjoying the taste of my food, and my sleep started to settle down.

19

The Six Tastes

Using the Six Tastes for Better Sleep

Ayurveda breaks down all food into rasa, virya and vipaka. Rasa is the primary taste, which is what we feel when we taste food. However, Ayurveda also speaks about vipaka, which is how a taste can change when it reaches the colon. An example of this is bananas. When we taste it in our mouth, it is sweet. However, it has a vipaka of sour, so it behaves like a sour food within our body. This influences elimination and detoxification.

In my family, there is a saying that on New Year's Day, you must make a relish for all the tastes. The philosophy behind it was that life is full of sweet and seemingly bitter situations, and you must embrace them all with equanimity and surrender to them. This is a beautiful concept. Ayurveda recommends using all six tastes in a meal as the best way to maintain balance. No taste should stand out. This is a simple way to bring balance into your meals and include ingredients that support better sleep. Avoiding a food item because you've developed a dislike for its taste is not beneficial to you.

The Six Tastes

Let us now look at the six tastes. The sweet taste is found mostly in carbohydrates, including grains, milk, fruits, some vegetables, in some fats and even in water. Many foods contain some sweetness, and it is quite a dominating taste on the tongue. It comforts your body and mind, and instantly relieves hunger. Keeping the sweet taste from fruits, vegetables and whole grains is beneficial. It calms excess vata and pitta. It is a cooling taste. Proper use of it supports building tissues and improving vitality, and is nourishing for the whole body. When it is in excess, it imbalances electrolytes, becomes a breeding ground for pathogens and promotes thirst.

The sour taste is fantastic in small amounts for digestion. Most sour foods, like lime, lemon, yoghurt and grapefruit, are helpful in digestion as they contain enzymes that help break down food. This also helps in elimination and detoxification. It is better to include this taste in moderation. For instance, add some lime juice in your food rather than drinking it as lemon water in the morning. Sourness is a heating taste. It calms excess vata. In excess, it causes digestive challenges, oedema, ulcers and excess thirst.

The salty taste is wonderful for electrolyte balance and adrenal support, if used the right way. Sodium–potassium balance is critical to so many other functions in your body. Salt is formed in water and exists in some foods like cucumber, celery and zucchini, as well as in mineral salts and aquatic plants. In small amounts, when used during cooking, it supports healthy agni, calms vata, maintains electrolyte balance, assists detoxification and softens the tissues. When it is too much, or when it is added after cooking, it causes imbalance to all systems.

The pungent taste of foods like onion, garlic, mustard, chillies, radish and spicy greens is stimulating. It helps fire up digestion and improves metabolism and secretion of enzymes. Many cultures which focus on prayer and meditation suggest avoiding this taste to slow down the system and calm down the mind. It is a heating taste. It decreases kapha, and increases pitta and vata. In moderation, it stokes the digestive fire, enhances absorption, aids circulation, assists with elimination of waste and clears the sinus. In excess, it causes fatigue, nausea, heartburn, insomnia and mental imbalance.

The bitter taste supports detoxification. It is found in many leaves like neem, lettuce, endive and arugula, as well as in aloe vera and turmeric, and in vegetables like bitter gourd. It helps detoxification and calms pitta when it is in balance with other tastes. It is drying and cleansing. It breaks up toxins, kills pathogens, supports the pancreas and promotes flavour. In excess, it depletes the tissues, causes dizziness, increases fatigue, reduces bone marrow, weakens agni and increases vata. Raw green smoothies can weaken agni, increase vata and disrupt sleep.

The astringent taste in also medicinal. It is said to heal the body because it dries up secretions. It is found in tea, spinach, okra, garbanzo, unripe bananas, alfalfa, turmeric, pomegranates and most legumes. It increases vata, and decreases kapha and pitta. In moderate amounts, it draws out toxins, improves the absorption and binding of stool and cleanses the body. In excess, it contributes to insomnia, anxiety, nervousness, poor blood circulation and a scattered mind.

When vata is in balance, the preferred tastes are sweet, sour and salty. When it is off balance, with weak agni, preferred tastes may switch to pungent, bitter and astringent. Predominantly, those with vata constitutions, vata imbalance and sleep challenges must have balanced meals. Consuming large quantities of bitter, pungent and astringent tastes further increases vata and disrupts sleep. Ensuring that no taste stands out in a meal will help maintain balance.

I mentioned a relish my family makes. It contains neem flowers for bitterness, salt, jaggery for sweetness, tamarind for sourness and red chillies for spice. The moment you eat a little of that, you salivate profusely, which helps with digesting any food you eat later. The next time you find yourself avoiding a taste, remind yourself to embrace them all so that you may also embrace all the flavours that life throws at you.

Using Taste to Support Sleep

Unless you have specific health challenges, such as being prediabetic, follow some basic frameworks to support optimal digestion and promote balance in all body systems. Sweet foods are nourishing for the body. In some amounts, so are salty and sour foods. Bitter, pungent and astringent foods are cleansing. We must keep them in balance unless there are special considerations.

Balancing the meal has great potential to support optimal sleep.

1. The right balance prevents imbalance and disease, and promotes health. Consuming an excess of cleansing foods, especially with high vata and poor sleep, can worsen problems. Excess sweet can cause problems when kapha is high, as in lymphatic and glymphatic congestion.
2. Whole grain consumption may vary based on constitution and state of balance or imbalance. Rotating them is the best way to stay in balance. They are mostly sweet, but do have bitter and astringent tastes. They include rice, wheat, amaranth, barley, buckwheat, millet, oats, rye, quinoa, jowar and bajra. In excess vata or with poor sleep patterns, you should initially minimize bitter grains like millet and quinoa. Choose whole grain options always. Aim to fill a quarter of your plate with them.

3. Legumes have some sweet, but are also bitter and astringent. They balance the whole grain. They are more drying, so eating them alone can increase vata and disturb sleep. Soak them for twenty-four hours, discard the water, cook them in boiling water, ghee and spices, and use them when digestion is strong. A reaction to them indicates weak digestion. See that their portion size is slightly smaller than the whole grain, but close to a quarter of the plate.
4. Animal proteins may replace legumes. Keep heavier forms of animal protein for lunch, when digestion is stronger. Fish is especially beneficial to good sleep.
5. Nuts and seeds are generally sweet, followed by bitter and astringent tastes. They are said to be building foods (help to build tissue), but because they are hard to digest, that can counter their benefits. They are most nurturing when cooked with food. In small amounts, they help vata as they are grounding, Nut butters tend to weaken digestion and increase vata.
6. All fats are primarily sweet and support balance of vata as they counter dryness. Consuming high-quality fats is essential to support agni, balance vata and improve sleep. They keep the nervous system calm. Using them, especially ghee, is beneficial. Ghee supports all constitutions, strengthens agni, calms vata, soothes the nerves and improves sleep.
7. Organic and grass-fed dairy calms vata, if you can tolerate it. In excess, it clogs channels. Consuming it warm or at room temperature is best. Cheese is not recommended. However, fresh milk, buttermilk and ghee are wonderful.
8. Spices aid digestion, especially when simmered in ghee before adding other ingredients to awaken them. Mineral

salt, coriander, turmeric and ginger together are a great combination to support better sleep.
9. Vegetables can be nourishing or cleansing. It is best to have one from each category to avoid agitating vata. Nourishing vegetables include avocado, beetroot, carrot, cucumber, Malabar cucumber, fennel, lotus root, parsnips, summer squash, yellow pumpkin, pumpkin, bottle gourd, ridge gourd, sweet potatoes, turnips, yams and zucchini. Cleansing vegetables include asparagus, bamboo shoots, beet greens, bitter gourd, bok choy, broccoli, Brussels sprouts, burdock root, green cabbage, purple cabbage, cauliflower, celery, Chinese cabbage, palak, methi, kale, mustard greens, arugula, endive, okra, peas, spinach and Swiss chard. Make sure vegetables complete the other half of your plate.
10. Fermented and processed breads are highly drying, so they imbalance vata and disrupt sleep. They draw out water from the system. Caffeine overstimulates the nervous system and raises vata. Alcohol deranges all constitutions, if consumed regularly or in excess.

20

Therapies for Your Sense of Taste

Use the nutrients and therapies provided in this chapter to keep your tastebuds balanced and improve your sleep.

Replenish Micronutrients for Mouth Microbiome and Taste

If you find that your problem lies with your gums, teeth or tastebuds, look into the supplements listed here. Avoid using these until you have done the work of cleaning up your diet and included the therapies from the ten-sense protocol, which is explained at the end of the book. Most often, things clear up with just that. Always consult a skilled practitioner before adding specific nutrients like these. It is important that the individual constitution is assessed.

L-tryptophan: Your body makes serotonin from tryptophan. Serotonin reduces with age. L-tryptophan works well because it helps to increase serotonin levels. Amino acids are used to make protein, but they also have so many other functions. It has been effective in treating insomnia.

Zinc: Zinc fights disease. If you have a bitter taste in your mouth, zinc deficiency could be the problem. Poor tastebuds and picky eating are both associated with zinc deficiency. Poor taste can make you aware of only salt and sweet tastes. Many metabolic enzymes require zinc. To have a healthy sense of taste, and to improve the quality of your sleep, supplement your diet with zinc.

Sadhana or Therapies

Oil pulling is a practice which has been handed down from ancient wisdom. It involves swishing oil in your mouth for a few minutes. Shown to restore bacterial balance, it cleanses your teeth and prevents gum inflammation, removes plaque, supports the health of your oral microbiome, reduces teeth sensitivity, restores healthy gums, promotes healthy sinus, removes tension in the jaw and helps to enhance your sense of taste.[93]

Here are the four simple steps of oil pulling:

1. Measure a capful of sesame oil. I add some turmeric powder as well.
2. Swish it around in your mouth for five minutes.
3. Spit the oil somewhere outside. Avoid spitting it into the sink or toilet as this may lead to clogging.

The Right Way to Clean Your Tongue

Tongue cleaning has also been a part of ancient wisdom. The health of your tongue can speak volumes about the health of multiple systems within your body. Tongue cleaning clears toxins from the tongue, removes the coating on the tongue which leads to bad breath, supports overall oral hygiene, improves the quality of the oral microbiome and enhances our sense of taste!

Look for a stainless steel or wooden tongue cleaner. Your tongue scraper may form a V shape. Place it towards the back of your tongue and move it forward while applying very gentle pressure seven times. This should clear debris and bacteria. Spit out any remaining saliva and wash your mouth with warm water. Repeat this seven times.

Studies have found that regular tongue cleaning reduces bacteria. Adding it to your brushing routine is best. It was also found that tongue cleaning altered taste perceptions and that can be beneficial for supporting your sense of taste.[94]

Sense Withdrawal to Soothe Taste

To restrain your sense of taste, incorporate fasting into your life. This can be challenging. First, start being mindful of whether you need taste and food all the time. Is being without food challenging to your body or your mind? Sit for a few minutes before you eat after breaking your fast and appreciate the food in front of you a little more. Think of those who struggle with finding food. Feel how grateful you are to have the food in front of you. Savour the taste of your meal and really appreciate it.

How Rahul Improved His Sleep Using His Sense of Taste

The migratory motor complex, or MMC, is an essential part of your digestive system and is responsible for cleaning undigested food, bacteria and anything else out of your gastrointestinal tract. It has a peristalsis movement, which travels likes waves right through your digestive system. It is very important to fast between meals for normal functioning of the MMC. When you hear your stomach growling between meals, it can just be your MMC working. The correct functioning of the MMC is important to maintain gut motility. Eating three meals a day, and not eating every two hours as is a popular recommendation nowadays, keeps the MMC working efficiently.

Rahul started to practise tongue cleaning and oil pulling every morning after brushing his teeth. He started humming while doing his suryanamaskar. He eats three meals and avoids eating every two hours. His meals are balanced with six tastes, always including a whole grain, a legume or animal protein, one leafy green, one sweet potato or another vegetable, ghee and spices. He kept a journal and eventually released his habit of eating in a rush. He makes his meal a sacred experience, and sits down and eats mindfully. He finishes dinner before sunset, giving his body time to feel calm and get ready to sleep. His anxiety came down, he enjoys his food and his sleep has restored itself beautifully!

PART 7

The Sixth Sense: Detoxification

21

Digestion and Detoxification

The karmendriyas are motor organs that perform actions and communicate. They play a role in the interaction between our inner and outer worlds.

In terms of the sense of excretion, the sense organ is your rectum, the final exit point of the digestive system. For optimal functioning, your liver needs to be working efficiently. All stages of digestion are intricately connected and cannot be looked at in isolation. Any hinderance in digestion, at any level, will impact detoxification. This is what is weak agni in Ayurveda, which impacts your sleep. This sense correlates with the sense of smell and is an earth element. Earth is stable, solid and resistant to change.

Genetic variations could also be a reason for poor detoxification, especially if these are associated with the health of your liver, the critical organ of detoxification. A history of antibiotic usage, overmedication, heavy food, poor eating practices, weak digestion, trauma that might inhibit detoxification, thyroid dysfunction, excess weight or weight loss resistance, candida overgrowth, a restrictive diet with nutrient deficiencies and anger could all be reasons for poor detoxification.

Sleep disturbances have been found in people with severe liver disease. Potential reasons could be the disturbed metabolism of melatonin and alteration in thermoregulation.[95] However, your liver can be a reason for poor sleep even in other cases. It is your liver that must metabolize and shunt out hormones after they have been used. Lack of optimal detoxification can be a major cause of poor sleep.

Liver Plays the Largest Role in Detoxification

Your liver is the largest organ in your body, located directly below the diaphragm on the right, under your ribcage. It has two major lobes, on the right and the left respectively. There are two more lobes on the rear. It's not important that you go deep into the anatomy of your liver, but it is useful to have an overview to understand how problems in your liver impact your sense of detoxification and cause problems with your sleep. Your liver purifies almost a litre and a half of blood every minute!

Those with liver problems have significantly more sleep disturbance than others. They take longer to fall asleep, sleep for a shorter duration, experience daytime sleepiness and poor sleep quality, wake up frequently in the middle of sleep and possess poor circadian rhythm, and low levels of melatonin.[96] While studies today only point to this connection in severe conditions, ancient Ayurveda recognized the connection between the liver and sleep thousands of years ago.

Detoxification Impacts Your Sleep

Keya had severe sleep issues. The doctor had put her on sleeping pills for some time. Initially, it improved her sleep, but, after a while, it started to get even worse.

She had been struggling with sleep for a few years and had started to believe that there was no way out for her. She was depressed. Her husband got irritated with how frequently she would talk about her sleep problems. As she was so exhausted, there was no intimacy between them. During the day, if they had even the slightest disagreement, she would end up uncontrollably angry or weep terribly. She constantly oscillated between anger and tears. She was trying her best to control it, but her emotions burst out. She thought she had become a bad person.

I asked her, 'Do you have regular bowel movements? Do you have any issues with your digestion?'

She replied, 'I have struggled with chronic constipation for many years. I take some fibre regularly. Sometimes it helps. Most times, it does not. I also forgot to mention that if I don't take the fibre, my skin flares up and I have haemorrhoids.'

She said that this contributed to her poor relationship with her husband as well, for when she had flares, it was impossible for her to have any intimacy in her marriage, and she felt it was her fault.

She said, 'In the last few months, I'm unable to sleep. I find myself waking up in the middle of the night with anxiety. Everything in my life looks super scary. At that point, I struggle to fall asleep.'

Her elimination was erratic. Was there any toxic exposure? Why was she not able to detoxify efficiently?

Understanding Digestion and Your Sense of Detoxification

Western science is only now discovering the powerful link between your gut health, state of the microbiome and sleep health. There is substantial evidence to show that the gut microbiome affects digestion and plays a role in regulating sleep.[97] There is plenty of research to prove that the microbiome in the gastrointestinal tract and gut is intertwined with the circadian rhythm.[98] A healthy gut also controls your mood, while an unhealthy one is implicated in anxiety and depression.[99] Mood disorders are also a root cause of poor sleep.

How Pitta Dosha Is Connected to Your Liver and Sleep

In Ayurveda, pitta dosha relates to all biotransformation. So, all of digestion is linked to pitta dosha.

Pitta dosha is responsible for all transformation in the body. The qualities of pitta are hot, oily, wet, sharp, light, subtle, flowing, hard, smooth, mobile and clear. It governs all chemical and metabolic transformation, digestion of food and mental digestion. Think of pitta as related to inflammation.

The functions of pitta include all aspects of digestion, regulation of body temperature, hunger, thirst, metabolism, hormone utilization, conversion of nerve impulses, creation of warmth and the ability to discriminate.

The primary home of pitta dosha is the small intestine. Additional homes of pitta include the stomach, sweat, blood, lymph and eyes. It produces acid and bile from the liver and small intestine.

Triggers of pitta imbalance include spicy or acidic foods, excessive heat, loud activities, aggression, excess competition in the mind, watching aggression, excess oily food, daytime napping, too much sun exposure, alcohol and caffeine. Notice how many of these interplay with triggers of poor sleep.

Other symptoms of pitta aggravation include acidity, inflammation, feeling hot inside, haemorrhoids, anger, inflamed skin, yellow sclera, burning eyes, difficulty sleeping and PMS. Once again, a lot of correlation to sleep challenges when pitta is imbalanced.

Someone who has a tendency to identify with the characteristics of pitta dosha, should set boundaries with work time, so they can avoid burnout and high stress.

Overall, pitta can be calmed down by soaking in cool water, avoiding overwork, focusing on relaxation, avoiding excess sun, cultivating playfulness, smelling sweet fragrances, including cooling herbs in the diet, drinking aloe juice and cool teas like hibiscus, maintaining a light yoga practice and practising yoga nidra. I discussed much of this in the section on touch in the context of histamine and pitta.

An Acidic Stomach Is the Best

Once food crosses your oral cavity, it enters your oesophagus, a long tube from your mouth to your stomach. Hyperacidity and gastro-oesophageal reflux disease (GERD) keep many people awake or give them disturbed sleep. Food moves down your oesophagus through peristalsis, which is a rhythmic wave-like movement of the smooth muscles. During this movement, there should be major mucus release to help lubricate the journey of your food.

Your stomach is a potent powerhouse that should be programmed to take care of many things for you. It must not only break down your food, but also destroy any pathogens that come with it. When your stomach receives food, it triggers HCL, or hydrochloric acid. When you try and stop the production of HCL in your stomach, it can cause a problem. If you have been prescribed antacids or proton pump inhibitors, remember that they might have been prescribed only for a short time. I see people staying on them for months and even years.

If you don't chew enough or only drink smoothies, you can severely impact your stomach acid. If you struggle with fungal infections, bad breath, diarrhoea, headaches, heartburn, sweating, foul odours, stomach problems, taking vitamins, indigestion, stomach pain, vomiting, skin conditions, anaemia, stomach infections or a desire to skip breakfast, you could have low stomach acid.

If you suffer from heartburn, then you are well aware of how it troubles you and prevents quality sleep. Heartburn, coughing and choking can prevent you from sleeping as they tend to worsen when you lie down. The backflow of acid from the stomach to your oesophagus can reach as high as your nose and throat. You might not feel the symptoms at times, yet it has been shown to physiologically disrupt your sleep.[100] When my heartburn was at its most severe, my nostrils felt like they were on fire. Sleep challenges and GERD commonly go hand in hand as they share risk factors. The bidirectional relationship is complex to understand with research, but this is evolving.[101]

Other than the fact that heartburn can wreak havoc on your sleep, low stomach acid and poor digestion can impact detoxification. Ample acidic chyme is required to stimulate the release of hormones, pancreatic enzymes and bile.[102] Detoxification is critical when it comes to all health and sleep. The section on agni in this book will bring an Ayurvedic perspective to digestive health.

What Happens in Your Small Intestine, the Home of Pitta Dosha?

Your small intestine is where nutrient absorption occurs. The carbohydrates start breaking down in your oral cavity, and proteins in your stomach. A tiny amount of fat digestion begins in the oral cavity through the release of lipase. But most fat digestion occurs in the small intestine via the release of bile. Your liver plays a critical role in your sense of detoxification. The small intestine is the home of pitta dosha.

Small, finger-like projections called villi in the small intestine walls allow nutrients to get absorbed. These villi can get compressed or worn down in autoimmune conditions like celiac disease, and in any condition where excess mucus and an irritated gut come together. Bowel inflammation and frequent parasitic infections can also cause damage to your villi. This is what leads to gut permeability or a leaky gut. When you eat something like gluten, if agni is weak, multiple things happen. Gluten increases a protein called zonulin, which is responsible for wedging itself in the tight gap junction of the small intestine villi and creating gaps there, leading to intestine permeability.[103] What this means is the molecules of food which are not as microscopic as they should be are absorbed into the bloodstream, where your immune system treats it is an invasion and launches an attack.

Some research has found that our immune system then gets confused, intestinal inflammation increases and your immune system is on high alert constantly.[104] As your villi gets worn down, and since different villi absorb different vitamins and minerals, you become deficient in many. You might not find research validating this connection, but it is common to see people have nutrient deficiencies when their gut health is compromised. The Ayurvedic perspective is that we need balanced agni to absorb nutrients from food. With intestine permeability, your blood brain barrier also becomes permeable, and science is finding correlations between the gut and the brain, especially in anxiety and depression.[105] Since the pituitary and hypothalamus are in the brain and control all your endocrine systems, it can finally impact any of the endocrine pathways and cause multiple events. Does this mean you must never eat gluten? I think not. However, it does require temporary elimination while working on optimizing digestion and detoxification. Once the system is in a state of balance, you should be able to eat heavier grains like wheat at lunch when agni is high, unless you have celiac disease or gluten sensitivity. It also depends on the source. Wheat in the US is highly contaminated and this makes it a problem for most people.

How does a leaky gut or intestine inflammation disrupt your sleep? Intestine inflammation keeps the levels of inflammatory cytokine elevated. Many studies have found that those who do not sleep well have elevated cytokines, which are immune system messengers.[106]

When you sleep poorly you risk dysbiosis in your gut. Poor sleep robs you of nutrients, makes blood sugar unstable and leaves you with a poor microbiome. Pathogenic bacteria like Prevotella can proliferate, in turn causing insomnia. Having a poor microbiome makes you more prone to poor sleep. Serotonin is critical to sleep and is linked to the gut microbiome.[107] GABA is a natural calmer and is also produced by gut bacteria.[108] Low GABA can correlate with anxiety and poor sleep. Gut microbiome diversity is associated with sleep physiology in humans.[109]

Can an Usually High Dose Vitamin D Make You Worse?

While speaking about gut health, emphasis must be laid on vitamin D. It plays a key role in several aspects of health, so it is important to look at it in some detail.

Vitamin D is a hormone that is essential for the absorption of calcium and phosphorus, healthy nervous and immune systems, regulation of hormones, normal cell growth, gut health, sleep and so much more. Low levels will impair immune functioning and are associated with many modern chronic diseases.

Vitamin D drops due to inadequate exposure to the sun, living in places that do not see the sun or living in cold or places of high altitude, inefficient production in your body, lack of vitamin D from your diet, using sunscreen or fairness creams, skin colour, liver health, kidney health, gut microbiome and much more that we may not know yet.

Vitamin D deficiency is associated with an increased risk for sleep disorders, poor sleep quality, short sleep duration and unhealthy sleep.[110] On the other side, poor sleep can also impact vitamin D levels and prevent your body from absorbing it optimally. You need optimal functional ranges of between 60–80 to promote good sleep.

Vitamin D in high doses challenges may impact sleep negatively. This is because vitamin D shares an inverse relationship with melatonin. I personally cannot tolerate a high dose of vitamin D, which is prescribed by many. I lose sleep and feel immensely agitated. I suspect that those with suboptimal liver function like me may be impacted more than others. My suggestion is to take a lower dose of vitamin D with fatty foods in the morning.

Vitamin D, Acetylcholine and Sleep

A study by Dr Stasha Gominak, who has been featured on my podcast, found that vitamin D might produce changes in the gut microbiome. She is the first to explain the link between vitamin D deficiency, sleep disorders and the abnormal intestinal microbiome. Gut bacteria need vitamin

D, and vitamins D and B favour the return of four specific species: Actinobacteria, Bacteroidetes, Firmicutes and Proteobacteria.

Dr Gominak explains, 'Maintaining vitamin D levels in a sleep-promoting range of 60–80 leads to increased deep sleep and more cellular repairs. The lack of microbiome supply of B5 paired with increased use eventually depletes body stores of pantothenic acid, causing reduced cortisol production, reduced acetylcholine production and increased arthritic pain and widespread pro-inflammatory effects. Pantothenic acid deficiency then decreases acetylcholine, which is the neurotransmitter used by the parasympathetic nervous system. Unopposed, increased sympathetic tone then produces hypertension, tachycardia, atrial arrhythmias and a hyper-adrenergic state known to predispose to heart disease and stroke.'[111]

22

Agni for Great Sleep

Agni is the fire element within us that is responsible for all transformation. It produces enzymes, assimilates nutrients, supports cellular communication, regulates temperature, provides energy, supports immunity, balances appetite, regulates blood pressure, supports elimination, ensures good sleep and is required for all health. When agni is weak, food is improperly digested, triggering accumulation of toxic waste and, eventually, dosha imbalance. *All health and good sleep depend on balanced agni.*

Agni is linked to how we digest our food and how we digest life. Our ability to cope with what happens around us is very much linked to how we digest our food. These are simple recommendations with age-old wisdom that have stood the test of time. Sticking to them prevents confusion over altering trends in diet recommendations. You can tweak the basic principles to suit you personally.

Healthy agni is supported by balanced meals. Including nourishing foods, like whole grains and sweet vegetables, and cleansing foods, like proteins, leafy greens and cruciferous vegetables, supports stable agni. Other ways to balance agni include:

1. Include all six tastes, balancing warming spices with cooling spices to support healthy digestion.
2. Use clean fats such as ghee, coconut, olive and sesame oil for cooking. Ghee supports all body constitutions. It lubricates the mucosa, is easy to digest and supports balanced agni.
3. Never add salt after cooking. Using salt while cooking allows for better digestion and encourages absorption of any water in the meal. Always simmer all your spices in the fats before you add anything else to awaken the spices and support healthy digestion.
4. Thinly slice or chop a quarter teaspoon fresh organic ginger. Add two or three drops of lime and a pinch of mineral salt. Have this before your meal. Antacids are never the answer.
5. Chew food until it is liquid. Avoid excessively watery foods which put the fire out. Avoid drinking any water with your meal.
6. Eat when you are calm. Be mindful and avoid all distractions which take away energy from digestion.
7. Eat only three meals a day. The modern trend of eating every two hours is neither local nor from ancient wisdom. Snacking is one of the biggest reasons for weak agni and high vata.
8. Eat food that is mostly warm and cooked for easy digestion. Anything cold weakens agni. In hot weather, stay with room temperature food.
9. Stick to a sleep schedule. Go to bed and wake up at a regular time.
10. Exercise. Focusing on abdomen strengthening movements can be helpful for long-term recovery from any digestive problem. Include yoga asanas like supine butterfly, warrior, sitting twists, gentle seated forward bends and triangle.

11. Feed your microbiome with prebiotics, probiotics, pectin, resistant starches and polyphenols. Many plant foods are prebiotic. I do not advice fermented foods as many people suffer from histamine intolerance. Resistant starches like oats, legumes, plantains and aloe can help to build a better microbiome. They resist digestion and reach your colon, where they are converted to short-chain fatty acids. These increase the growth of good bacteria.[112] Pectin from stewed apples feed beneficial bacteria. Warm cooked apples with ghee and spices at breakfast can calm vata. Avoid combining fruit with other food as they digest at different times and can cause digestive distress.

My Healing Digestion course helps you understand the source of healthy digestion, root causes of imbalance and the foundational principles of optimal digestion using functional medicine and Ayurveda.

23

The Liver and Detoxification

Your liver is the critical organ of detoxification. Your colon and rectum are the exit points which allow excretion to happen. Your liver is also the seat of your anger, according to traditional Chinese medicine and Ayurveda.[113]

It's crucial that your liver works efficiently as it detoxifies you, produces cholesterol, stores and converts glycogen to glucose when required, stores minerals and fat-soluble vitamins, eliminates metabolized hormones, protects you from parasites, neutralizes poisons, metabolizes alcohol, discharges waste and regenerates its own tissues. Digestive distress, constipation, skin issues, low energy, obesity, headaches, anger, jaundice and poor sleep can be signs of liver dysfunction.

When poor liver function impairs your blood sugar balance, you may end up waking up at night. Elevated liver enzymes increase insulin resistance and impact blood sugar stability.[114] When it creates hormone problems, it can prevent oestrogen from being metabolized, leading to oestrogen dominance, and causing insomnia and interrupted sleep.

If liver dysfunction is impairing digestion, it can cause heartburn and constipation, both of which can create problems with sleep.

Every nutrient and toxin that enters your body must pass through the liver before it enters the blood for circulation. It is the main site for poison control as it detoxifies, breaks down and purifies so that nothing harms you.

The first phase converts toxins to metabolites. In the second phase, these same metabolites are merged with a molecule which can allow them to leave your body via different pathways. If one of those pathways gets congested, toxins accumulate in fatty parts. When excess fat builds up on your liver itself, it leads to a common condition known as fatty liver disease. Imbalance in pitta is why fatty liver occurs.

Antacids, antibiotics, poor gut bacteria, fluoride, low levels of iron, zinc and vitamin B, selenium, toxins, petrol fumes, chemicals, hair dyes and anything toxic can inhibit these pathways.

If your liver does not release a steady flow of bile, bile can also harden in the ducts of your gallbladder, causing gallstones, which then lead to immense pain and even gallbladder removal.

What Is Methylation?

Methylation controls gene expression. Your genes might make you predisposed to specific behaviour and influences your physiology, psychology, appearance and proclivity for certain diseases. A gene mutation is a permanent alteration in the DNA sequence and can affect anything from a single DNA to a large segment of a chromosome that includes multiple genes. Your genotype is the set of genes in your DNA which is responsible for a particular trait. Your phenotype is the physical expression, or characteristics, of that trait.

Methylation is a series of biochemical pathways that breaks down nutrients from food, gut and cells. Many processes like genetic expression, conversion of food to energy, cellular protection, brain health, production of neurotransmitter hormones, stress response, detoxification, immune response, cardiovascular function and DNA repair take place here.

It is a part of both phases of liver detoxification. Most of the nutrients required for the phases to function properly are created in methylation pathways. If someone has a genetic variation which prevents proper methylation, then their body might be depleted of certain nutrients like folate, B12, some amino acids like tryptophan, magnesium, choline and zinc. The same deficiencies can also cause problems in methylation.

In the conversion of food to energy within your cells, you create free radicals. High levels of oxidative stress slow down systems. Methylation will not work in this stage.[115]

If you do not methylate properly, then you do not make enough melatonin, and when you do not sleep properly, then you do not methylate properly. This is a vicious cycle.[116]

How does methylation and detoxification impact each other? Chemical or toxin exposure is overwhelming. If you struggle to deal with a huge burden of toxins, then your genes will try to compensate wherever possible. Then, methylation will be affected. If you have poor methylation, then your detoxification will be poor as well. There is another vicious cycle. If you do not detoxify, then you will elevate the stress hormone cortisol.

Methylation pathway detoxifies oestrogen, dopamine, histamine and heavy metals. They need magnesium to function. Toxic substances combine with a methyl group and then go out of your body via a pathway. Nutrients like choline and B vitamins activate these detoxification pathways.

What Is COMT?

The Catechol-O-methyltransferase (COMT) gene plays a key role in the metabolism of catecholamines, oestrogen and neurotransmitters. When there are some genetic variations in the COMT gene, you could have problems metabolizing catecholamines, leaving you in a perpetual state of fight or flight.

It also is dependent on a healthy methylation cycle.[117] The role of genetics in healthy sleep is attracting more interest and research. Variations in the COMT gene may have critical effects on vulnerability towards poor sleep and sleep quality.[118] Even if you have a COMT variation that predisposes you towards poor sleep, it will help you tremendously to support the health of your liver, prevent oestrogen dominance, keep yourself free of high-stress triggers that release catecholamines, improve detoxification and elimination, have plenty of exercise to help burn off excess catecholamines and observe if caffeine is a problem for you. Focusing on all that prevents you from slipping into a state of sympathetic dominance, or fight or flight, will be deeply supportive. The DNA Company does wonderful work in sleep genetics.

Supporting Your Liver to Improve Sleep

I've heard so many people tell me that their friends ridiculed them for stressing over sleep troubles. It's usually followed by the friend flippantly telling them that they have had sleep troubles for years, or even decades, and they end every night with alcohol followed by a sleeping pill. The reason you feel that a glass of wine helps you unwind and fall asleep is that moderate alcohol helps to initially promote sleep.

Alcohol causes some blood sugar imbalance. When you go to bed you may trigger a blood sugar drop during sleep, which initiates a cortisol spike followed by you waking up or having restless sleep. This can also increase insulin resistance.

Studies have shown that there is a connection between alcohol and sleep. It can have either a stimulating effect that impacts sleep onset negatively or it can have an initially sedative effect which helps you fall asleep, but may not be long-lasting. It can also impact REM, sleep continuity and total sleep time based on how much and how often you drink. It was also found that late-afternoon drinking also disrupted sleep, suggesting long-lasting changes in sleep regulation.[119] If you are struggling with sleep, avoiding or reducing alcohol may be necessary. Combining alcohol with sleeping pills can be very dangerous. Alcohol is also dehydrating, so it increases vata. It is also a pitta-aggravating trigger.

Alcohol can also mess with hormones and increase oestrogen dominance. Since alcohol is also a load on your liver, which is the primary detoxification system, it can impact liver function. The subsequent suboptimal liver function can be another reason for oestrogen dominance. If you want to enjoy that glass of wine, do so occasionally and in moderation along with a balanced meal that can create a buffer.

How Do You Support Your Liver to Improve Sleep?

1. Begin by following all the practices for healthy digestion and keeping agni strong.

2. Avoid late-night snacking. Your liver rejuvenates between 11 p.m. and 4 a.m., and you need to be in deep sleep during that time.
3. Reduce your exposure to toxins. Reach for organic foods, drink purified and clean water, avoid using the microwave, stop colouring your hair, switch to perfumes made with essential oils, stop using shampoos with parabens and reduce every kind of toxic exposure. Also reduce the use of non-stick cookware, aluminium, air fresheners, perfumes and pesticides.
4. Vegetables like beetroot are especially supportive to liver health. Bitter foods can support liver health, but overdoing them without balancing other tastes can also cause problems. The key is to include them at all meals, in balance.
5. Add a bitter herb like triphala to support liver detoxification. Start with half a teaspoon twice a day mixed in hot water before food.
6. Reduce your levels of stress. If you find a situation or a person particularly stressful, either avoid it altogether or find ways where you can feel disconnected to the stress of the situation.
7. Reduce anger. Find ways of releasing and letting go. It also helps to do guided meditations from my podcast while lying on the ground.
8. I've saved the very best for the last. Castor oil packs can be the game-changer. I describe the benefits and methodology at the very end of this section.

Understanding the Colon, Home of Vata Dosha and Sleep

Your large intestine, or colon, plays a crucial role in digestion. It absorbs any final nutrients, including fluids and some minerals.

This is also the area of your digestive system where bacterial colonization is at the highest. Bacteria play a critical role in the absorption of key nutrients.

Excretion is as important as nutrient absorption. Vata aggravation is why constipation occurs, so anything to combat the dry quality of vata prevents constipation.

With chronic constipation comes the elevation of cortisol, oestrogen dominance, poor methylation, poor sleep and waking up unrested.

Fibre is the critical component of excretion and detoxification. Fibre is found in plant foods, so no matter what your diet, it's important that you consume enough plants. It also supports metabolizing hormone metabolites.[120]

Fibre can be soluble or insoluble. Soluble fibres like oats, lentils, pectin and psyllium husk hold water and can be soothing and gentler on digestion if you struggle with gut sensitivity. It can dissolve in water or hold water and leave through your gastrointestinal tract. It can also help to soothe the gut when it is inflamed. Insoluble fibre like vegetables can irritate when you do not have enough fluids.

If you have symptoms of constipation, which include a lack of daily bowel movement, straining to eliminate, dark coloured or hard stool, frequent headaches or poor sleep, check your diet and see if you need to change something. Avoid foods that are cold, raw or dry, which increase vata dosha.

Rectum Health, Haemorrhoids and Sleep

In terms of the sense of excretion, the sense organ is your rectum, the final exit point of this entire digestive system. Problems in your rectum can create immense pain. Keya had mentioned her haemorrhoids to me at the start, and the more I worked with her, the more I saw how miserable it made her.

Haemorrhoids are swollen blood vessels in and around the anus and lower rectum. They occur when you stay chronically constipated for years.

The squatting toilet of olden days was supportive to elimination, and the posture of squatting itself supports blood circulation in the hip area. Challenges with elimination was unheard of in the era this was practised, at a time when people's diets were free of processed foods. Poor blood circulation and lymphatic movement in the pelvis as a result of sedentary lifestyle is also a reason for haemorrhoids.

Having a look at the emotional aspects of release can improve detoxification. Learning to let go and release emotionally and mentally supports physical release and excretion. In the same manner, improving your elimination physically, can start a process of emotional and mental release.

Specific Protocols to Improve Constipation

1. Squat! Sit for a while in a squat every day to bring blood flow to the hips and improve elimination. If you find it tough to squat, squat and lean against a wall, but stay there for two minutes.
2. Explore journal writing and see what you are holding back or not releasing in your mind. Holding on to a grudge or bitter feelings sets destructive patterns and makes you hold back physiologically as well.
3. Drink warm fluids to keep vata calm. Tea, coffee and alcohol do not count. In fact, they increase the amount of fluid you

will require to counter their effects. Do not consume any fluids with your meals.
4. Drink aloe juice on an empty stomach. The mucilaginous aloe creates a slippery coating through the colon and helps other fibres move through easily. Use fresh aloe or juice without any preservatives. You can also apply aloe gel topically and locally for haemorrhoids.[121]

24

Therapies for Your Sense of Detoxification

Therapies and nutrients in this chapter are specifically for improving digestion and overall detoxification. Many of these therapies are already a part of the ten-sense protocol.

Replenish Micronutrients to Improve Detoxification

Aloe Vera

Aloe vera is a miracle in calming pitta imbalance. If you grow aloe vera in your garden, just cut a stem and remove the flesh to make juice. Have this on an empty stomach every morning until symptoms reduce. If you do not have access to fresh aloe, look for aloe vera juice without preservatives. Aloe is a natural laxative which works without causing a strain on physiology, unlike other laxatives. It also stimulates mucous secretion.

Triphala

Triphala is a tridoshic herb which supports digestion and detoxification. It is especially effective for vata imbalance and helps all constitutions in moderation. It is best to mix half a teaspoon of triphala powder with a half teaspoon each of ghee and honey, unless you are prediabetic and cannot consume honey. Used with these carriers, it is warming. To be more cooling, you could mix it with aloe vera juice. Do not start with it if pitta is very high. If it tastes bad, you need it. If it tastes fine, you do not.

Sadhana or Therapies

These are powerful therapies to support detoxification, so use them cautiously. Overuse can be dangerous and detrimental. I have used them cautiously in the ten-sense protocol in the best ways possible to be of benefit to you. The reason I bring caution is that I see a lot of people overuse these therapies and then suffer tremendously. Please use them only as I have advised or consult a skilled practitioner.

Enema

Enema is an age-old practice to improve detoxification and can be very supportive if done occasionally and with some precautions. Through the right kind of enema, digestion can be improved at every stage, from nutrient absorption to excretion. Enemas done too frequently can weaken the colon. It is best to do them under supervision, or once or twice as part of a therapeutic protocol. In this case, my advice is to do an enema once to get the body healing. It is better to reach out to an Ayurvedic centre for basti if you are keen to explore deeper healing. Basti is a better option, where the colon is nourished with herbs and oils.

You can buy a home enema kit, fill it with warm water and a little salt. Insert the tip into your anus and hold the canister at a higher level for water to flow in easily with the help of gravity. Eventually, when the whole can of water enters your colon, remove the end from your anus and sit on the toilet. Another word of caution is to be very careful after an enema as the microbial balance can change, making you susceptible to infections. If done once, it can help sleep.

Any medical questions regarding contraindications and cautions, or any questions on whether one is to proceed with enema as provided above should be referred to qualified health professionals.

Castor Oil Packs

Castor oil has been used traditionally in my family for generations! Even as children, we were given a little castor to consume every so often as it was my great-grandmother's regular practice to keep the digestion system clean.

External castor oil packs are my most favourite tool for sleep. They decrease straining during defecation and reduce symptoms of constipation.[122] They help your body with complete evacuation and can be as effective as a laxative. Castor oil packs can improve glutathione production. Glutathione is a master antioxidant, but can be weak in people with health challenges. It plays a key role in liver health and detoxification.[123] What I have found personally is that they help me activate the parasympathetic nervous system and calm down a hyper mind.

Apply a palmful of castor oil over your liver area. Your liver is under your right ribcage. Wrap an old cloth around your midriff and tie it with a soft cotton tie. Wear an old shirt and leave it on all night, or let it remain for an hour or two and then wash it off. If you are a woman, avoid them when you have your period. For specific castor pack recommendations, work with our programme.

Sense Withdrawal to Soothe Detoxification

To restrain your sense of detoxification, try to restrict indulgence and modify your diet to one that is supportive to elimination. As you start to eliminate, you also start to release emotions that do not serve you. This might feel challenging, but as you feel the benefit, you will also start to understand that the rewards are more important than the feeling of restriction. Food that serves you need not taste bad. Try to explore immensely flavourful preparations that also serve detoxification.

Gut Microbiome and Sleep

The Gut Microbiome and the HPA Axis

The relationship between sleep and the gut microbiome is bidirectional. Sleep deprivation causes significant changes to gut microbial composition, which may lead to gut barrier dysfunction and inflammatory cytokine production.[124] Similarly, gut microbiome and inflammation are linked to sleep loss, circadian misalignment and mood disorders.[125] Most strikingly, preliminary evidence suggests that gut microbes and host circadian genes interact with one another. In fact, gut microbes have their own circadian rhythms, just like humans. For example, Clostridiales, Lactobacillales, and Bacteroidales, which account for 60 per cent of total gut microbiota, experience rhythmic fluctuations that mirror the host's biologic clock.[126] The gut-sleep relationship can be explained by examining key biological mechanisms.

The HPA Axis

The HPA axis is a system that mediates the effects of stress on the immune and nervous systems. It is activated by psychological stress and inflammation, stimulating the release of cortisol from the adrenal glands. Cortisol is a neurohormone associated with stress, and it is also acts like an internal alarm clock. Cortisol levels surge in the morning to help wake us up and get us out of bed. Unsurprisingly, consistent activation of the HPA axis and the associated cortisol release can affect sleep quality and duration. The gut has a strong influence on the inflammatory state of the body, and consequently impacts HPA activation and sleep.[127]

Leaky Gut and HPA Activation

The gut microbiome is populated by several bacteria, including both gram-positive and gram-negative bacteria. Gram-negative bacteria have a cellular membrane comprised of lipopolysaccharide (LPS), which is released into the gut as these bacteria die. While in the gut, LPS is mostly benign and gets excreted through faeces without causing any problems to the host. However, when the gut barrier is damaged, LPS can seep into portal circulation, leading to systemic inflammation and nervous system dysregulation.

LPS can affect the HPA axis in two different ways. First, it stimulates the production of inflammatory cytokines which interfere with cortisol receptor signalling. These cytokines dislodge cortisol from its binding sites, sending them into the bloodstream and dramatically increasing serum levels of cortisol. Secondly, LPS binds to adrenal cells directly, which stimulates additional cortisol production.[128]

Improving Sleep by Leveraging Gut Health

The gut barrier can become damaged through excessive antibiotic use, diets high in saturated fat and artificial ingredients, emotional stress, illness and other causes. Addressing these factors is ground zero for tackling gut-related sleep disturbances. However, a more robust, targeted approach is often required to fully restore the gut barrier. Probiotics, prebiotics and other gut mucosal-support products are ideal options for aiding gut barrier function, regulating the gut–brain axis and improving sleep parameters. There are several probiotics available on the market, but only a select few are clinically shown to target biomechanisms related to sleep. For example, certain Bacillus spore-forming strains, such as the novel strain B. subtilis HU58™, are found to reduce inflammatory cytokine levels by up to 50 per cent and may also reduce serum cortisol levels.[129] These functions can help calm an overactive HPA axis, and may support sleep quality and duration. Similarly, a novel strain known as B. longum 1714 is clinically shown to improve sleep quality and duration, particularly in subjects undergoing stressful situations. The proposed mechanism of B. longum 1714 is like that of Bacillus spore-forming probiotics. For example, 1714 can reduce

> concentrations of inflammatory cytokines, lower cortisol output and elicit a calming response in the nervous system.[130]
>
> Kiran Krishnan
> General Manager, Novozymes OneHealth North America Microbiome Labs

How Keya Improved Her Sleep Using Her Sense of Detoxification

Keya took the foundational steps to have a strong and stable agni seriously. She included castor packs several nights a week, which were miraculous in helping her shift her sleep. When she felt a little better, she did just one enema to help her detoxify on a deep level. The first thing she noticed with the castor packs was a huge change in her mood. She no longer had uncontrollable anger or frustration. She felt better than she had felt in a long time. Her sleep started to settle and she got her life back.

There are specific tests which when elevated indicate folate and B12 deficiency, liver challenges and methylation issues. Please schedule a consultation with us for specific details on labs, analyses and recommendations.

PART 8

The Seventh Sense: Uro Reproduction

25

The Urinary System and Vata Dosha

The sense organ of uro reproduction is the genitals. It allows you to urinate, experience sexual pleasure and procreate. If you have any issues with the urinary system, then it can keep you up or keep waking you up through the night, disrupting sleep. There is a strong relationship between the kidneys and the adrenals as well. Sexual gratification and good sleep are linked, especially as it connects to oxytocin flow. Healthy ovulation is required to stay calm and sleep well. Healthy fertility supports a calm brain. This sense correlates to the sense of taste and the element of water. Water represents fluidity and flow, and allows life to exist.

This chapter mainly explores a woman's body, except for the sections on prostate gland health and general recommendations. The reason for this is that it is mostly women whose sleep is impacted by problems in the reproductive or urinary system. Lack of sleep at different times of the month can make coping with your day a struggle. Hormone supportive recommendations can apply even to men with symptoms like frequent urination, hot flashes and sleep disruptions.

In Women, Hormones Can Be a Symphony

It's amazing how many women speak about cycle-related sleep disruption. Your hormones should gently ebb and flow like waves on a calm day. The menstrual cycle impacts circadian rhythm and sleep.[131] Premenstrual sleeplessness, disturbed dreams and fatigue are often reported. This can impact the quality of life.

Hormones help maintain all health as they are chemical messengers between systems. They regulate mood, metabolism, hunger, growth and sleep. The relationship between hormones and sleep is one more bidirectional axis.

How Is Uro-Reproductive Linked to Poor Sleep?

Jenny struggled with sleep and experienced severe insomnia at specific times of her cycle, along with feeling exhausted at other parts of her cycle. She had been treated repeatedly for urinary tract infections until urine culture reports showed that no antibiotic had been effective. She did not have excessively heavy cycles, yet she struggled with PMS symptoms, and oscillated between anger and tears. She had no libido and did not enjoy intimacy with her partner. Most of all, the lack of sleep at different times of the month made her struggle to cope with a day filled with managing her little son and keeping up with work. It was destroying all aspects of her life.

Jenny had been struggling for years and had started to believe that all women felt the same way. 'Is there a way out? I've started to feel so dejected at the state of my health, my sleep and even my life!' she told me.

We found that she was dealing with severe oestrogen dominance and low progesterone, had many inflammatory signs and recurrent yeast infections which started with any sign of intimacy.

She had gained a lot of weight in the last ten years. She was too tired to exercise and dragged herself to the gym, where she did some heavy training. Jenny mentioned having a few abortions before her son was born. She drank tea or coffee all morning to cope with the routine of getting her son to school and racing to work. She had frequent sweet cravings that became unbearable in the evening. She usually succumbed to pastries or cookies at that time. She also carried headache medication in her bag all the time, for she never wanted to struggle with her recurrent blinding headaches when they came unannounced.

Before her period, her breasts were swollen and tender, and hurt when someone hugged her. Her clothes became tight and she looked visibly bigger. People started asking her if she had gained weight, which depressed her even more, especially at a time when she was so emotionally sensitive. She lost sleep. One thing I noticed was her hair. It was a golden brown, and when I asked her if that was her hair colour, she said that she coloured her hair every week.

Your Urinary System

Challenges that many women and men face with their urinary system negatively impact the quality of sleep. The reason that women struggle with more challenges is simply because of anatomy.

If you have any problems related to your urinary system, be it an infection or an irritable bladder, then you are naturally torn between drinking enough water to be less in agony but needing to wake up through the night as result versus not drinking enough water and waking up in agony. Symptoms are temporarily relieved by drinking water and then become worse since it can mess up sleep altogether. If you have vata aggravation, excess water can weaken agni and further imbalance vata.

Women have a very short urethra, which is the connection between the bladder and the exterior of the body. This makes us prone to infections.

There are many urinary challenges that can impact your sleep. When Jenny struggled with her symptoms, at first it was repeated bladder infections, which can be utter misery. If you keep treating these infections with antibiotics, or self-medicate for bladder infections, then it impacts your entire microbiome, including your vaginal microbiome, putting you at risk for yeast infections.

Breaking the Vicious Cycle of Bladder Infections and Poor Sleep

Bladder infections in women inflame the urethra and the bladder.

What causes these infections? Using public toilets when you are sensitive to these infections is a major risk factor. Neither can you not use them, since these infections can make you feel such an urgent need to urinate that you are ready to use any restroom. When you keep getting bladder infections, then you keep using antibiotics, which are required to clear up the infection, but also can be the cause of further infections since they destroy the microbiome. Poor circulation in the pelvis is also a trigger.

What can really be troublesome for recurrent bladder infections is sexual contact. You're probably torn between wanting to avoid it altogether to save yourself from that horrendous feeling and dejection that this is destroying your relationship.

What happens in bladder infections is that a bacterium which is present in the body is in the wrong place and has grown to pathogenic proportions. The reason for this can be that the colon is close to the bladder and vagina, and excessive friction or lack of fluids can change the pH, causing inflammation and growth of pathogenic bacteria. Sometimes, other bacteria like Klebsiella and Staphylococcus also cause bladder infections.

Also, many of the underlying causes of poor sleep, such as cortisol action, sympathetic nervous system response and immune dysfunction, also contribute to bladder issues, which in turn impact sleep.[132]

Incontinence Impacts Sleep

Urinary incontinence is referred to as a leaky bladder. This can be a nightmare. When you are with people, it can upset your self-esteem and cause humiliation.

Before I explain how incontinence impacts your sleep, let me add some context:

1. Incontinence occurs in a situation of bladder stress, which can be caused by giggling, coughing or jumping. Weakening of your urethra or sphincter from frequent constipation can also cause challenges.
2. Poor sleep and urinary challenges have the potential to become a bidirectional axis. Vata aggravation is linked to poor sleep and frequent urination. It helps to begin with safe practices that calm vata dosha.
3. All forms of urinary incontinence can impact sleep as they can cause urinary leakage and discomfort during sleep, causing you to wake up. Different forms of incontinence can impact sleep in different ways. Sleep disturbance and fatigue are common for people with overactive bladders. In fact, they are associated with more severe bladder symptoms.[133]

Is It Possible to Sleep with Prostate Issues?

In the early embryonic stage, the tissue that becomes the womb in women and prostate gland in men is the same. The prostate gland covers the first part of a man's urethra and is located just below the bladder. Its main function is to secrete fluids that nurture the sperm, but many challenges in this area for men impact urinary function and sleep.

Symptoms of an enlarged or inflamed prostate gland can be linked to urinary challenges such as frequent urination, a burning sensation on urination, dribbling, urine retention and the subsequent risk of bladder infections. Chronic inflammation, vata aggravation and certain nutrient deficiencies may be reasons for men developing prostate gland issues. Increased testosterone and oestrogen can cause enlargement of the gland.[134]

An enlarged prostate gland can be a trigger for poor sleep. The narrowing of the urethra can prevent the complete emptying of the bladder, making you feel like you want to urinate more frequently and putting you at risk for bladder infections. Each time you wake up, you end up trying to urinate, not emptying the bladder, going back to a disturbed sleep cycle, only to wake up again when you feel like urinating. When you keep doing this, you also imbalance vata dosha, and it gets harder and harder to fall asleep again.

Calm Vata for a Balanced Urinary System that Supports Sleep

Some easy steps for your urinary recovery can include:

1. Foods that can cause bladder inflammation are caffeine, dry foods, airy foods, chocolate, alcohol and histamine foods, which are listed in the section on touch.

The Urinary System and Vata Dosha

2. D-Mannose helps urinary infections and bladder inflammation, but only if it is an E. coli infection. If you have frequent urinary infections, especially related to E. coli, antibiotics can make the problem worse. D-Mannose works wonderfully to treat bladder infections if you take it as soon as you feel symptoms. A word of caution though: You cannot keep taking it. Have caution using it if you are diabetic or prediabetic. Always consult your doctor.
3. Support liver health and detoxification. If the liver is not working optimally to clear out exogenous and endogenous toxins, then heavy metals like mercury can affect the mucosal lining of the bladder itself. It can also lead to histamine elevation and that can trigger bladder irritation. This also goes back to having strong agni and healthy digestion.
4. Address trauma. Trauma that impacts the pelvis can keep muscles in a state of tension. Relaxing the pelvis can release trauma, improve blood circulation and increase lymphatic flow in the pelvis.
5. Cranberry can help. Most cranberry juices in the market are also high in sugar and feed bacteria. However, cranberry can prevent E. coli from sticking to bladder walls. Look for supplements.
6. Use a sitz bath to relax the pelvis. This is my all-time favourite therapeutic addition, as it not only helps you physically, but there is also something immensely calming and emotional about sitting in that warm water. Make sure the tub allows you to sit in water up to your waist. Add tea, herbs or essential oils to the water.
7. Assess fluid intake at night. It will help to drink more fluids during the day to maintain the bladder's detoxification capability, prevent night-time bladder irritation and restore some level of circadian rhythm.

8. Calm vata dosha. Vata aggravation impacts urinary patterns and sleep. Keeping vata calm supports healthy agni and lowers inflammation. I would always advice beginning with practices that support agni and balance vata before trying anything else.

26

How Hormones Impact Sleep

It's startling how many women speak about cycle-related sleep disorders. Most women can predict that they are about to ovulate or get their period by how messed up their sleep gets just before these phases begin.

An average menstrual cycle can be anywhere between twenty-seven to thirty-five days. Each month, a follicle starts to grow. Think of it as the source of all your hormones. Within this follicle, there are some that produce sex hormones. After a week, the most dominating follicle is chosen. It grows bigger and bigger while the other follicles disintegrate. Only the healthiest egg will then mature and the rest get reabsorbed. The maturing follicle sets off a release of oestrogen which thickens the lining of the uterus. This is in preparation for fertilization. The rising oestrogen triggers the pituitary gland to release LH, our luteinizing hormone. This triggers ovulation, where the ovary releases a mature egg. It moves into the fallopian tube hoping to be fertilized.

Within your ovary, there remains a section of your ruptured follicle. If the egg is not fertilized by a sperm in the fallopian tube, what remains of the ruptured follicle within your ovary becomes active again. It becomes a yellow gland-like substance called the corpus luteum. Your corpus luteum grows for ten days until around the twenty-fourth day of your cycle, at which point it starts to disintegrate. Between days fourteen to twenty-four, it produces significant amounts of progesterone and oestrogen. This production of hormones is what causes the endometrium to thicken, preparing to receive a fertilized egg. If there is no fertilization, then the endometrium sheds, triggering a period.

To understand why this impacts sleep, I also need to take you through what happens in other parts of your body. Menstruation and ovulation are completely dependent on a communication axis, knows as the HPG axis, or the hypothalamus pituitary gonad axis. There are two hormones produced in your pituitary gland. Follicle stimulating hormone, or FSH, encourages the follicles to release their egg, leading to ovulation. It makes oestrogen rise. When oestrogen is higher, your hypothalamus receives a signal and triggers your pituitary to release luteinizing hormone, or LH, which causes ovulation to occur. In the first two weeks, or your follicular phase, LH is low. When oestrogen reaches its highest, LH also rises and then drops again. In the first part of your cycle, oestrogen starts to rise and then drops. In the second part of your cycle, progesterone is released and oestrogen also rises. When your period approaches, both fall sharply, causing PMS and your period.

Oestrogen and progesterone are both required. They also need to be in balance with each other. Oestrogen, in its good form, helps insulin resistance, promotes growth hormone which has multiple benefits, keeps your mood stable, regulates hunger and provides you with stable energy. Progesterone balances oestrogen. It is produced after ovulation in the luteal phase. It is soothing for the brain, supports good sleep, stimulates thyroid hormone and makes you feel calm.[135]

What does oestrogen do for you in your body? It helps with skin health, heart health and blood flow to the brain. It creates the endometrium and increases fat; it is responsible for fluid retention and can trigger depression when it is not in balance with progesterone. It is also the culprit for those terrible hormone headaches. Imbalance can also cause poor sleep. Progesterone, on the other hand, helps you use fat for better energy rather than storage. It is a diuretic and allows you to pee out retained fluid.[136] It can also prevent hormone headaches, and it promotes sleep! Yet, many women are put on oral contraceptives for hormonal migraines, which can be detrimental.[137]

Oestrogen dominance, which so many women struggle with, can be caused either by having too much oestrogen, not being able to get rid of oestrogen metabolites or having low progesterone. If you have low progesterone, you can have sleep symptoms such as insomnia, restless sleep and frequent waking. Oestrogen dominance can happen due to excess weight, a diet that is high in starch or sugar, not having a gallbladder, liver congestion, stress, exposure to environmental oestrogen in the form of xenoestrogens of plastics and parabens, and phytoestrogens in the form of soy, meat and dairy. If you've been on birth control pills, that can cause oestrogen dominance as well.

Why does your sleep fluctuate with your menstrual cycle?

1. Progesterone is required to relax your body and calm your mind. Research suggests that low progesterone, such as in perimenopause, can impact sleep.[138] If you have low levels of progesterone, then you will struggle with sleep towards the end of your luteal phase and experience PMS. Progesterone also increases GABA and serotonin, and therefore, low progesterone can impact mental health and sleep.[139]
2. Low progesterone with oestrogen dominance can affect sleep. Low iron, which can be the root of hormonal imbalance, also causes restless legs which impacts your sleep.[140] If you have

conditions like polycystic ovary syndrome (PCOS), where you do not ovulate regularly, then low progesterone can affect sleep. Progesterone in the luteal phase, which is the second half of your menstrual cycle, can work in different ways. It can be sleep supportive since it is calming and promotes sleep. But progesterone also causes your core body temperature to rise in the luteal phase, which is a pitta phase.[141]

Let's look also at how specific sleep challenges occur through the menstrual cycle.

During the menstrual phase, there is a drop in oestrogen and progesterone that can trigger sleep challenges. It can also make you feel less rested even if you seemed to have slept. The reduction in iron levels can also impact sleep, triggering sleep issues such as restless legs, migraines and chronic fatigue. If you are generally sensitive to hormonal shifts, then this phase can be a major trigger for poor sleep. Menstruation is also a vata phase and any vata imbalance can trigger poor sleep. It is also common to find sleep challenges closer to ovulation. The phase up to ovulation is a kapha phase, one that makes the body cooler. One reason could be that women are less aware of sleep impactful environmental issues like temperature and noise when more fertile.[142] One interesting study indicated that in ovulation, women slept less if they had more attractive partners.[143] During the late luteal phase closer to your period, you could have sleep challenges as a result of the temperature increase from progesterone and the drop in melatonin levels. Cooling practices can be supportive. It can also be due to falling oestrogen and progesterone levels in preparation for a period. Luteal insomnia is a sign of vata imbalance.

You should begin tracking when you are losing sleep the most. In the first phase of your cycle, which is known as the follicular phase, oestrogen starts to build up and then falls closer to ovulation. In the luteal phase, which is the phase from when you ovulate to when you get your period, progesterone rises. If you've had optimum ovulation, it is sleep supportive until PMS. Increased core body temperature was observed in the mid luteal phase.[144] In the first part of the luteal phase, sleep might be great once progesterone is released, but then it starts to reduce in the mid luteal phase.

Studies have also shown that there are significant changes in REM sleep due to the menstrual cycle. The menstrual and circadian cycles are also connected.[145]

What you can do to support sleep if you have problems in the luteal phase is to try and keep your core body temperature low by cooling yourself with food and baths. Remember this is a pitta phase. Then, progesterone will work for you and promote good sleep. You may also face the other problem of feeling too sleepy in the luteal phase. You may experience sleep issues at ovulation. There is some argument that this may be connected to ancestral adaptation and fertility, as studies point towards women with more attractive partners sleeping less.[146]

It's important to maintain a sleep diary and track the days you lose sleep. Then, you can begin to understand what you need to do. In the hormone steps I've curated for you, I've specifically divided it into follicular support and luteal support so that you can optimize your hormones to support sleep much better.

How Stress Messes with Your Hormones

It's essential to understand the connection between stress and progesterone as it plays a crucial role in good sleep. The first thing to understand is the link between stress and ovulation. Progesterone is produced after you ovulate. When progesterone is released, it has a connection with GABA, a neurotransmitter hormone that makes you feel less anxious.[147] This is also the reason that when progesterone starts to drop towards the end of the luteal phase, tipping into PMS, you lose sleep, feel extremely anxious and have a horrible time coping.

If you have high levels of stress, you stay in fight or flight, which is what is vata aggravation. High vata has the quality of excess dryness. It counters what we require for healthy hormones. High vata from stress weakens agni.

Your body is programmed to react to high stress by shutting off non-essential functions such as immunity, reproduction and digestion.[148]

Overexercising is a trigger of vata imbalance. The body thinks it's a fight-or-flight situation and is unsure what to do. So, if you are running marathons every week or training hard, you might just not produce progesterone.[149] You may not want babies, but you do need progesterone, nonetheless.

The other aspect of this connection between stress, progesterone and sleep is that it is a vicious cycle. If you don't get optimum sleep and are low in melatonin, then it will impact how you produce progesterone as there is a synergistic relationship between the two.[150]

Navigating Menopause and Sleeplessness

Perimenopause is a vata time of life. Progesterone starts to decline and drops more rapidly than oestrogen. This is a time when oestrogen dominance is very common.

At that age, oestrogen dominance can create uncomfortable symptoms such as depression, hot flashes, fluid retention, headaches, insomnia, palpitations, night sweats, incontinence and tearfulness. So many of these symptoms can disrupt sleep in many ways.[151] Perimenopause can last close to a decade. During perimenopause, it's as if your brain does not remember many basic functions such as temperature regulation and circadian programming.

Since progesterone controls mental calmness, emotional balance and healthy sleep patterns, low progesterone and an oestrogen dominant state in perimenopause instantly causes all forms of sleep disturbance. If progesterone keeps fluctuating and is not optimal, it impacts production of GABA. Ovulation can be non-rhythmic and even missing at times during this phase.[152] This affects how much progesterone is produced.

Menopause also causes hot flashes, which happens due to the hypothalamus and pituitary being preoccupied with managing so many other changes. Hot flashes are immensely upsetting for sleep. Intertwined with body temperature elevation, it leads to uncomfortable night sweats.[153]

What you can do right away is find ways to reduce your core body temperature, which includes soaking in a cold-water tub once for ten minutes or avoiding forms of exercise that are immensely heating.[154] A safe and gentle way to maintain the right body temperature is practising abhyanga several times a week.

Since menstruation can be frequent, heavy and with heightened PMS symptoms, those can be disrupting to sleep as well. It's common to see women waking up through the night to change a tampon or empty a menstrual cup. Excess bleeding is a sign of excess pitta, which impacts sleep.

If you have excessive bleeding that is keeping you awake at night, while that might be a part of perimenopause, also be mindful that other factors such as iron deficiency anaemia and oestrogen dominance can also cause it. Sometimes, addressing anaemia with adequate iron from food sources and supplements, if necessary, can reduce excessive bleeding. You could also have scanty bleeding, erratic cycles and poor sleep, which are all symptoms of vata imbalance.

Can You Have Great Hormones that Support Great Sleep?

Let's look at some easy steps for hormone recovery before we go into the section on the role of sexual health and intimacy on sleep.

1. Eat an anti-inflammatory, hormone-boosting diet.
2. Restore the circadian rhythm. I urge women wearing a dark eye mask when they go to sleep.
3. Balance blood sugar. Blood sugar balance and hormones are two sides of a coin.
4. Prioritize exercise, but avoid overtraining. Explore gentle forms of exercise like yoga, tai chi, walking and swimming. Swimming lowers core body temperature. Yoga calms down your autonomic nervous system. Walking helps to move the lymphatic system.
5. Avoid any restrictive diet.
6. Avoid alcohol. It not only puts a strain on your liver, but also impairs the early sleep phase, where the growth hormone is released.
7. Support liver health. When you are constipated, oestrogen metabolites can stay in your body, making your body more oestrogen dominant. Constipation is a major reason for hormone disruption. Also avoid the triggers of vata aggravation.
8. Be specific about protocols and therapies with phases. If you have tracked your sleep through your menstrual cycle and

notice any specific times when you are impacted, try to use supplements and therapies based on the root cause. Read the section where I have listed out the specific root causes for poor sleep at different phases of your cycle. For example, if you struggle with sleep during the late luteal phase due to temperature elevation, do a cold-water soak or daily abhyanga to regulate temperature. If you struggle with sleep at ovulation due to LH spikes, it might help to support brain health with a head massage before dinner.
9. For perimenopause, support reduction of hot flashes with half a cup of aloe juice. Drink coconut water or hibiscus tea to cool down from within.

If you follow the protocols and still have trouble with your hormones, please seek a qualified practitioner who can run specific hormone labs and do what is necessary. Deep hormone work is beyond the scope of this book.

27

Sexual Energy and Vitality

Air, water, food, sleep, and sex are vital to human survival. There is evidence that suggests sexual suppression is a big factor that can contribute to inflammation.[155] You know how suppressing your emotions can be inflammatory. Sexual suppression is similar to this.

Good relationships are crucial to support healing and recovery. Similar to how being with someone who makes you laugh and relax is powerfully healing, sexual happiness also supports your body in so many ways. When sexual suppression is high, there is limited oxytocin release and pent-up emotions. This could lead to deep stress, increase in cortisol and higher inflammation since the release of oxytocin and decrease in cortisol are both crucial players in reducing inflammation. Oxytocin decreases cortisol and improves resilience to stress.[156]

Sexual satisfaction has been linked to better immunity.[157] C-reactive protein, or CRP, produced in your liver is elevated under inflammation. Studies have shown sex can be beneficial in lowering inflammation.[158]

Sexual suppression can cause immense pelvic stress. A strong pelvic floor is associated with higher rates of sexual activity.[159]

A strong pelvic floor is always helpful, especially for women, in bladder and reproductive health. If there is active sexual suppression and subsequent tension stored in your pelvis, it can contribute to aggravation of bladder issues and pelvic pain. In yoga and traditional Chinese medicine, emotions and the pelvic area are innately connected. Tension in the pelvis can create tension in the mind as well. Ancient wisdom advises that sex should neither be suppressed nor overused.

28

Therapies for Your Sense of Uro-Reproduction

Can You Use Temperature to Soothe Hormones?

Urine is the best reflection of your core body temperature, which is deeply linked to good sleep. Soaking in a tub of cool water rapidly lowers your core body temperature and reduces even concerning urinary symptoms like burning, discomfort and the tendency towards bladder inflammation.

Basal body temperature is the temperature of your body first thing in the morning. Oestrogen influences blood flow, vasodilation and heat dissipation, and lowers core body temperature. Progesterone does the opposite. Reproductive hormones have important influences that can significantly alter your thermoregulatory response.[160] During the follicular phase, your temperature can be anywhere between 36.11 to 36.4 degrees Celsius. After ovulation, it rises progressively and can rise about two-tenths of a degree until it reaches a plateau. It then stays elevated at that temperature until menstruation begins.[161] My suggestion would be to track your basal body temperature for one full cycle at the same time every morning. Note the days where you lose sleep. This will immediately offer you insights on how to use therapies to help sleep.

Replenish Micronutrients for Your Urinary and Reproductive System

Vitamin B6 plays a key role in hormonal health. It is required for progesterone production. It is also needed for protein metabolism, formation of red blood cells and a healthy immune system. It supports energy production, as well as the production of adrenal hormones. It helps in liver detoxification and enhances REM sleep.

Sadhana or Therapies

Feminine Sitz Bath

Sitz baths bring blood circulation to the pelvis, relax internal muscles and allow for more movement in the area.

You require a tub which can hold water and allow you to sit so that the water comes till your waist. Fill the basin with warm water. Boil some tea. Add it to the water. When you finish, lie down for a while and bring your awareness to the sensation of blood flow through the pelvis. Feel yourself releasing and letting go.

Cold Water Therapy

Cold water therapy stimulates the vagus nerve. Stimulation through cold water also results in higher HRV.[162]

Soak in a tub of cool water for ten minutes. Your core body temperature will regulate much better and you will finish feeling better than when you started. Do not do this too often. When the body feels overheated, use it as a therapeutic tool. You do not need to soak in ice soak. The cool water from your tap is sufficient.

If you include some warm oiling before a bath daily, it can be beneficial to sleep. Warm water can help with sleep. Remember to listen to what your body needs. Ayurveda is all about opposite brings balance.

Sense Withdrawal to Soothe Your Reproductive System

To restrain your sense of uro-reproduction, go for a walk outside or include some spiritual practice every day for a few minutes. Walking in nature lowers cortisol, is grounding, improves lymphatic circulation, which is crucial to your urinary and reproductive system, and helps detoxification. Incorporating a spiritual practice such as meditation is considered a wonderful way to support this system as well.

How Jenny Improved Her Sleep Using Her Sense of Uro-Reproduction

Jenny first worked on steps to strengthen agni, and calm vata and pitta, focusing on warm and moist foods. She drank a quarter cup aloe juice thrice a day for a month to help hormone regulation. She noticed by tracking her sleep that the worst times were in the luteal phase for her. She did a cool soak to help her regulate her body temperature. Afterwards, she focused on daily abhyanga for optimal temperature regulation. She stopped going to the gym and joined a yin yoga class, focusing on calming down her body and mind. She noticed herself feeling more stable. Her PMS went away, and her sleep has become easier and deeper. She feels gratitude for all that is going well in her life and uses journalling to release any pent-up emotions.

PART 9

The Eight Sense: Locomotion

29

Locomotion, Movement and the Circadian Rhythm

Your legs symbolize many things, primarily the ability to move. They represent your journey, in a way, and your ability to take yourself from one place to another, both physically and symbolically. I want to take you through something very interesting to make you understand how your legs play a major role in your balance. If you've ever practised yoga, think about when you stand on two legs and when you stand on your head. In a headstand, with your arms forming a tripod, you have a larger surface area of your body in contact with the floor, as compared to your two feet when you are standing up. Yet, its common to feel unstable in a headstand and the opposite when you stand on your feet. Why is that?

Your legs symbolize balance in all forms, including the balance between your two sides. Using your legs, you can move from place to place and experience locomotion. Your legs also symbolize feeling grounded and feeling connected to the earth, bringing with it a sense of stability and rootedness. The sense of locomotion is a fire element, which allows us to experience movement and radiance. It correlates to the sense of sight. Fire, or tejas, allows for light, perception, radiance and movement.

Movement allows you to release cortisol and feel balanced emotions. It lets you release anxiety and increase BDNF, allowing new brain cells to grow and protect your brain.[163]

Do We Hold the Key to Longevity?

Lympha is the Roman deity of fresh water. She is connected to the god of fountains and water, and she represents a functional use of fresh water. Water is always thought to be fresh only when it is flowing.

Lymph is milky white, resembling Lympha. If your blood and your cardiovascular systems are active, your lymphatic system is your passive drainage system.

In Ayurveda, lymph is called rasa. This is the first of seven dhatus, or tissues, feeding subsequent tissues. What is fascinating is that the study of the lymphatic system is considered the study of longevity! I'm going to take you through the lymphatic system, rasa, kapha dosha and what a critical role it plays in your sleep quality.

How Locomotion Impacts Sleep

Luke struggled with sleep and experienced severe insomnia, oscillating between sleeping too much and staying wide awake, tossing and turning through the night. He had anxiety and fatigue, which he never faced before, despite a high-pressure job. His stomach felt uncomfortable, tender and painful. He was smoking a lot more than usual. He had little energy and nothing seemed to pick him up in the morning, not even a cup of coffee. He felt overpowered by fatigue.

Luke had been struggling with this for a year. He said, 'My wife is badgering me that I don't spend enough time with the family, but when I get home, I am so tired that I just sit on the couch to unwind, watch some TV with my dinner and fall asleep on the couch itself.'

I asked Luke if, in the last year, there had been any change to his lifestyle. He told me that he used to run, swim, do yoga and lift weights until his job got hectic, and he didn't want to add more stress to his day. Along the way, his daily movement reduced to a few times a week and now he was lucky if he managed a walk around the block with his dog.

Movement supports healthy digestion, immunity, healthy endocrine function, cardiovascular function, lymphatic drainage, a healthy hormonal system, a balanced and stable neurological system, apart from several other profound positive health benefits.[164]

Understanding Your Lymphatic System

The lymphatic system returns interstitial fluids to your veins and maintains fluid balance.[165] Without it, all your cells would be sitting in their own waste and bacterial debris, without oxygen or circulation. Lymph is collected from your lower body into lymphatic vessels and your muscles transport lymph through a one-way system leading up to your torso. There are lymph nodes throughout your body. These are in your armpits, groin, breasts for women and the throat. Most fat absorbed from your small intestine is too large to move through your blood. It first moves through your lymphatic system, which why your lymph is fatty.

It is comprised of mainly water and some protein squeezed out through capillaries.

Your lymphatic system removes fluid around tissues, filters toxins, transports white blood cells to areas that call upon them, helps absorb fat and subsequently transport fatty acids, and returns interstitial fluid back to your veins.

It is considered the most important system in Ayurveda. Rasa is the blood plasma and is related to kapha dosha. It provides nourishment and is responsible for the hydration of tissues, electrolyte balance and immune function. It is the most important dhatu, or tissue, as it nourishes all subsequent tissues. Not chewing your food enough, having weak agni, overeating, eating too often, going to bed or exercising before food is digested can impact rasa dhatu. The result is swollen lymph nodes. Nutrition from food and drink is refined and passed from rasa to the other six tissues.

Think of your lymphatic system as a distribution network for your immune system, protecting you from various bacteria, virus, fungi and pathogens. Lymph nodes can get swollen due to an infection, inflammation, lymphatic congestion, lack of exercise, cancer or some autoimmune condition. Once your lymphatic system has cleaned up your immune system, most lymph returns to your bloodstream. It is important to understand, though, that unlike your circulatory system, your lymphatic system does not have a pump to do the job. It requires gravity, pressure and movement to circulate lymph.

The Impact of the Lymphatic System on Your Body

The lymphatic system has many subdivisions and problems can arise in any of them.

Gut associated lymphoid tissues (GALT) are a concentration of lymph tissue in your gut. Much of your immune system is situated there, which is why gut health is at the centre of everything else![166] Among the signs of lymphatic congestion in the GALT are poor digestion, digestive symptoms of any kind, constipation, belly fat and a tendency towards developing haemorrhoids. GALT plays a key role in gastrointestinal disease.[167]

Mucosa associated lymphoid tissue (MALT) is a cluster of lymph tissue in all the areas where you have mucosa or wet tissue.[168] This is found within your respiratory, digestive, urinary and reproductive systems. Some of the signs that you have lymphatic congestion in your MALT are digestive problems caused by consuming wheat or dairy, digestive distress, bloating, nausea and fatigue.

Bronchial associated lymphoid tissue (BALT) are lymph tissues in your respiratory system.[169] Some of the signs that you have lymphatic congestion in your BALT are sneezing, congestion, colds, cough and heavy headaches from sinusitis.

Skin associated lymphoid tissues (SALT) are lymph tissues in your skin.[170] Some of the signs you have lymphatic congestion in your SALT are acne, hives, urticaria, eczema, psoriasis, dry skin, toenail fungus and fungal overgrowth.

The glymphatic system is a concentration of lymph tissue in your brain.[171] Signs you have glymphatic congestion include brain fog, waking up feeling low, anxiety, depression, mood imbalance, sadness, worry, poor memory, inability to focus and trouble sleeping.

General lymphatic congestion signs can be swelling and oedema, or a proclivity for both, being overweight, tendency towards water retention, swollen ankles, cellulite, fatigue and depression.

Liver's Role in Your Lymphatic System

Your liver produces a large amount of lymph, which can be as much as 30–50 per cent of what flows through your thoracic duct. Some observations link the lymphatic vascular system to liver diseases.[172] Lymphatic congestion can play a major role in liver challenges.

Most fat absorbed from your small intestine cannot directly flow through your bloodstream. Your liver must metabolize the fats and first move it through the lymphatic system. Your liver is the filtration system for all toxins and food. It also produces so much of your lymph.[173]

What this means is that the amount of fat that you eat plays a role in how much lymphatic movement is required;[174] the health of your liver and the health of your lymphatic system are connected, and how you digest fats is connected to the functioning of your lymphatic system.[175]

Love Your Lymph to Help Your Sleep

Let's explore some ways to look after the lymphatic system.

1. Deep breathing and breath work are some of the most powerful ways to get your lymph moving, even with more serious challenges.[176] Yoga can also be a wonderful way to move your lymph, especially when you have a practice which is complete with inverted poses, forward bends, backward bends, side bends and twists.
2. Apply castor oil on your liver area, and all the areas of your lymph nodes and your colon. If you add a hot water pack to these areas, you'll encourage lymphatic flow.

3. Have fun rebounding. Jumping on a trampoline can be so much fun. If you jump raising your arms and clapping each time, you'll add more power to get that lymph moving. Avoid this if you have signs of excess vata.
4. Dry brushing helps some people. If you have signs of vata aggravation, avoid dry brushing even if you have read that it is the way for lymph movement. Abhyanga with bath powder is far more potent.
5. Saunas can help some people. It will not work if you have histamine issues or pitta imbalance. We are all unique.
6. Cold helps many. When you put your body through this kind of stress, it finds resources to heal itself in ways it may not have done before.[177] However, if you have vata aggravation, the cold can make it worse. In that case, begin with gentle interventions like castor oil packs. It is also better not to overdo using the sauna and cold dips.
7. Colon hydrotherapy or an enema can shift things. Unloading the liver and colon can be a great way to improve lymphatic movement. Research found that it can improve colon and immune system function.[178]
8. Pomegranates are even better as they are potent phytonutrients for reducing inflammation![179] This should not mean overdoing just the astringent taste, but including it in your diet while maintaining balance.
9. Reflexology can help if you have had skin issues, especially something like toe fungus. You can really move that lymph along with reflexology or even just a good old foot massage.
10. Ayurveda knew the wise power of massage from ancient times. Apply some oil and move your lymph around as much as you can by yourself! Warm sesame oil is wonderful, unless you are in a hot place in the summer.

11. Walking works wonders. Even though I have mentioned walking last, I swear by it. Fast walking can be immensely helpful for lymph drainage. I speak about walking in detail later as well.

30

Movement for Great Sleep

How Does Your Sense of Locomotion Help Sleep and Longevity?

As I have said before, you are the pump for your lymphatic system and you support it through gravity, pressure and movement. Movement has been linked to benefits for all systems in your body, but especially for brain health. Movement releases BDNF, which behaves like a growth hormone for your brain and supports sleep for brain recovery.[180]

Exercise and movement play a major role in health, alongside sleep, relaxation, nutrition, hydration, stress and resilience. Through clinical practice, I've found that no matter how perfect someone's diet is, if they miss out on movement, they struggle.

Movement, or moderate exercise, supports healthy digestion.[181] Regular movement can strengthen your digestive system and improve elimination. It speeds up your metabolism, allowing you to use food for energy, and can decrease any digestive symptoms as well.

Oxidative stress occurs when you produce more free radicals than you can neutralize during the metabolic process of converting food to energy within your cells. Movement counters the effects of ageing by combating mitochondrial dysfunction, and by adding antioxidant and anti-inflammatory actions. Movement mitigates mitochondrial ageing and interrupts the vicious cycle of oxidative stress.[182] Cellular function is directly linked to the state of digestion. Ayurveda talks about agni being critical to cellular digestion. Combining movement with optimal digestion is key.

Movement releases the brain neurotransmitter hormones of beta-endorphins, dopamine and serotonin. As you know, serotonin is the precursor to melatonin and is important in the context of sleep—both to help you sleep and keep anxiety low.[183] Movement can also improve your circadian rhythm.[184]

Movement initially increases core body temperature and later allows it to drop lower, making it more conducive to falling asleep. The caveat though is that vigorous exercise can increase core body temperature and prevent sleep. What you must note is that if you do have a day of vigorous exercise, then make sure that it's not late in the evening, where you risk raising core body temperature and impacting the quality of your sleep.[185]

BDNF is a protein that supports existing neurons, and encourages the growth and differentiation of new neurons and synapses. In the brain, BDNF is active in your hippocampus, prefrontal cortex and forebrain. It improves neuronal function, neurogenesis, is neuro protective and helps with neuro plasticity. Neuro plasticity is extremely important as it allows nerve cells in your brain to compensate for injured ones or to deal with a new situation. BDNF triggers slow-wave sleep and the more sleep deprived you are, the more of it you need. Low levels of BDNF are associated with anxiety and depression. Think of it as the link between movement and emotions.[186]

Movement decreases time taken for sleep onset, which is the ability to fall asleep. It increases sleep duration, preventing interrupted sleep.[187]

How Ancient Wisdom Codified the Perfect Tool: Yoga

Yoga harnesses the specific power of inversions to support your lymphatic system. Dr David Haase, MD, a Vanderbilt-and Mayo-trained physician, and author of the bestselling book, *Curiosity Heals the Human*, says if the anterior cingulate is dysfunctional, and if there is frequent dysfunction in that area, then there is also a dysfunction in mood, attention, sense of self and more.[188] This is also where the gut and the brain intersect. My instinct got me thinking naturally of the area where the anterior cingulate and the path of yoga might cross. I thought of inversions, headstands, pranayama and more, and then I thought of meditation. Research is now looking more closely at the benefits that come from several ancient tools like pranayama.[189]

The second way yoga supports your lymphatic system is through muscle contraction. Think of sitting in a forward bend, holding your toes. When you stretch your large muscles, think about what happens when you stretch a rubber band. The more you stretch a rubber band, the greater the force with which it contracts and springs back when you let it go. Similarly, when you stretch your large muscles, the more you stretch, the more the muscles contract when you let go, allowing them to work like a pump, pushing blood and lymph back to your heart. There is something fascinating that happens when that blood reaches your heart. Your heart is fooled by that extra volume of blood into thinking that you might have done some aerobic movement and pumps stronger, sending fresh blood throughout your body. In this way, when there is muscle contraction through stretching, you support lymphatic drainage through a gentle form of movement.[190]

Finally, when you incorporate abdominal movement through spinal twists, lateral bends, and forward and backward bends, you allow lymphatic movement through the whole trunk of your body. Dynamic flow sequences like sun salutations and flow yoga allow lymphatic movement to occur through a curated sequence that connects movement with breath. Breathing is another powerful way through which you replace the missing pump in the lymphatic system. It can improve the quality of your sleep. Think of breathing as the movement of energy.

Yoga is an exercise which can be both gentle and vigorous. When it comes to sleep, my suggestion is to incorporate a gentle sequence with inversions and stretches towards the evening. If you want to have a vigorous sequence, then breath work might end up activating you and preventing sleep. In that case, it might work better to practice vigorously in the morning, when raising cortisol is beneficial in several ways. Vigorous and quick movement disrupts vata and imbalances the nervous system.

Walking, Lymph and Sleep

Walking was a part of ashram life for me. Silent walks through the forest and up the mountains seemed challenging. I did struggle and there were times I felt like hiding somewhere. I am glad the habit of walking was enforced during my ashram days as it made me realize its profound benefits. Quite recently, I started to track my sleep with different modalities and I discovered something amazing when it comes to walking. My deep sleep doubled on the days that I walked long distances. While researching this I found that walking improves the time taken to fall asleep, the duration of sleep and sleep quality![191]

I tracked my steps and distance rather than the time that I spent on walking. I made a conscious effort to increase it every week. For me, 10,000 steps could be covered in about 7 kilometres, and 20,000 steps in about 14 kilometres. Obviously, this may be different for you. Make sure that as you increase the distance you also compensate with recovering foods such as protein and antioxidants. Also make sure that you give yourself a day of rest and stretching after a day when you pushed yourself harder. If you struggle with sleep challenges, and you are still in the healing phase and, just starting to apply the protocols from this book, avoid running, which can be stressful to the adrenals. Be gentle yet firm in your approach. There is no one that you should compare yourself to. In the beginning, avoid trying to increase distance while reducing time. Even if it takes you more time to walk 10,000 steps, that is fine. Find a time of the day when you are free from responsibilities and dedicate it to walking.

Lack of Movement and Its Impact on Sleep

Sleep impacts your ability to incorporate movement and how much you move impacts how you sleep. Exercise has been a factor in good sleep for a very long time and is being found to hold a lot of promise as a non-pharmacological factor in supporting better sleep.[192]

Incorporating any movement in the early morning or afternoon can support setting a right sleep-wake cycle. Doing vigorous movement later in the evening or at night might upset the sleep–wake cycle in some people. For most people, it does not negatively impact sleep if exercise is moderate and stops about 90 minutes before sleep.[193] However, in this research study I am referring to, only men participated, and women can be more sensitive to these effects. If you find that you can only take time out in the evening, make sure that you do not engage in a vigorous form of exercise. Gentle movement like yoga, walking, swimming, or tai chi may support better sleep.

Restless Leg Syndrome (RLS) and Sleep

The fatigue created by lack of sleep can increase symptoms of RLS. In turn, these symptoms can prevent sleep. It is a condition where your legs are restless when you try to sleep. You start to feel an uncontrollable urge to keep moving or stretching the legs. Symptoms tend to get worse at night and hinder sleep. Common reasons for RLS are iron deficiency,[194] pregnancy, alcohol, caffeine, magnesium deficiency, hormonal imbalance and vata imbalance. It can also be due to lack of movement and stretching as well, which can lead to inadequate blood flow to the legs. Some medication such as antihistamines can also be a reason. Medication need not be the answer, though. Lowering overall inflammation and improving nutrition can also be very helpful. Check your iron status. Ferritin levels should be optimal, between 60–80. Yoga can also be immensely supportive as it stretches the fascia, and improves circulation and lymphatic movement.

Bringing in Movement into Your Life to Help You Sleep

It can feel challenging to be consistent with movement. There are times when we have too much going on. However, there are several ways you can bring movement into your day. You can solve any sleep problem if you put yourself first.

Building Your Movement Routine

1. Enjoy whatever magical triad of movement you choose. Yoga, swimming and walking are my magical triad, which I complement at times with strength training.
2. Merge movement with nature. Walking 10,000–20,000 steps is a great form of exercise to try and include a few times each week.
3. Think of movement like water. One of the things that I always teach at yoga is the five elements. When I talk about water, I speak about yoga practices like vinyasa, which bring together movement and breath work, where the priority is on the gracefulness of the transitions, rather than the pose itself. It teaches you to enjoy the journey of life, rather than focussing on the destination. Whatever movement you bring in, adding subtle breath awareness and feeling the grace in your movement makes it soothing and calming.
4. Movement that is gentle is powerful. Movement need not be vigorous, strenuous and aggressive. In fact, gentle and moderate movements can be far more effective as a tool to support better sleep as it calms vata dosha.
5. Movement should be curated specifically for you. Often, I find clients being pushed by trainers because their spouse is at a different level, leaving them in a constant state of physical stress, chronic fatigue and inflammation, which instantly affects their sleep. You are precious and you need a sequence designed just for you. Listen to your body constitution and speak its language to anyone who guides you in movement therapy.

31

Therapies for Your Sense of Locomotion

If you find that your sleep problems lie with your lymphatic system or your legs, or are a result of a lack of movement, then you need to explore this chapter in greater depth. If you face challenges with energy levels and struggle with exercise, it could be due to low iron or ferritin levels. It may be worth checking your iron levels and supporting your body so that it can start to exercise.

Replenish Micronutrients for Your Lymphatic System

Iron is vital for energy production, and blood cells low in haemoglobin due to iron deficiency can make you feel exhausted! Without iron, energy production is severely impaired, and chronic fatigue and exhaustion can occur. Iron functions in the production of cellular energy and metabolism. It is utilized in the formation of myoglobin, a red protein, which carries and stores oxygen in muscle cells and transports energy. Never take supplements such as iron unless it is recommended by a qualified health professional. Test, don't guess.

Sadhana or Therapies

Inversions

Using gravity is a powerful way of moving your lymph. One of the best ways to boost your yoga practice is by adding a headstand and shoulder stand. You can only do these if you do not have high blood pressure. Both postures support lymphatic movement and rest the circulatory system by allowing your veins to return blood to your heart without your heart actively pumping.

The headstand stimulates your pituitary gland, which is the master of your endocrine system.[195] It allows you to drain lymph in individual organs within your body, restoring better circulation to them later. I never advice trying these exercises by watching a video or as part of a large class where you might not get individualized attention.

The shoulder stand is gentler and passive, yet powerful, in moving lymph. It regulates the thyroid and parathyroid, helping metabolism and detoxification. Combining these two postures, along with the required counter poses for each, is one of the best ways you can support your lymphatic system and sense of locomotion.

Seated Forward Bend

A seated forward bend, with your legs together, holding your toes, is a way to use the power of muscle contraction to move the lymph. It also calms your mind and restores your ability to sleep.

If you can get your head to rest on your legs, focus on deep abdominal breath work, where you stick out your abdomen with your inhale and let it relax with your exhale. The pressure that it exerts stimulates lymphatic movement in the abdominal region. The seated forward bend should not be practiced if you have a prolapsed or slipped disc.

Sun Salutations

The mistake that is commonly made while performing sun salutation, or suryanamaskar, is how fast it is practised, with no deep breath work and no focused postures. Remember that the sun salutation is one of the best reminders of flow. It is a movement sequence that links together graceful transition with the right breath work. Allow yourself to breathe slowly and deeply, coordinating each transitionary movement with the required breath. The transition should be graceful and fluid, reminding you about the all-important journey rather than the destination, which is the philosophy of the sense of movement.

A practice of fifty-four or 108 sun salutations is a powerful lymph mover, but should only be done rarely, while maintaining a slow pace with focused breath work. I've seen social media challenges of 108 every day for ten days, and people going through it fast. All that does is aggravate vata.

The last thing you need with disrupted sleep is 108 suryanamaskars.

Barefoot Walking

Barefoot walking connects you to the earth, and is rooting and grounding.[196] Walking barefoot allows you to experience wonderful feedback from your feet, as well as become aware of your structure and your gait as no shoe can ever allow you to. It has an acupressure effect on your whole body. Extra cushioning in shoes can prevent you from using the right muscles.

You will also feel the ground better, and have much better structure and balance. It allows your feet to breathe. There are also many benefits such as better-developed and stronger leg muscles.

Sense Withdrawal to Soothe Your Locomotion

To restrain your sense of locomotion, sit in a cross-legged pose, or lotus pose, every day for some time. This can be challenging. Your knees may hurt and your back may feel uncomfortable. You do not have to struggle that way, but sitting quietly and binding your legs for a little while every day will allow you to really appreciate your ability to move.

How Luke Restored His Sleep Using His Sense of Locomotion

Luke found his magical movement triad in tai chi, walking and swimming. The tai chi class introduced him to a community of people who were also on a search for ultimate peace. Walking gave him solitude, an opportunity to reconnect with his true self, without goals or pressure. Swimming made him regulate his body temperature, which helped his sleep. He also focused on strengthening agni, his source of all energy. As his agni improved, the iron levels improved as well. His is now able to fall asleep easily and is deeply grateful to wake up each morning feeling radiant and motivated!

PART 10

The Ninth Sense: Grasping

32

Grasping, Strength and Nerves

Another bidirectional axis is that of pain and sleep. Pain is associated with sleep disturbances for many. Poor sleep quality in turn makes pain worse.[197] Pain is linked to inflammation and the health of your nerves.

The sense of grasping through our hands allows us to receive, gather, collect and hold. While we are focusing on the specific relationship between your hands, inflammation and pain, this chapter is a bird's-eye view to all inflammation and pain, and how they are linked to sleep.

> **Did you know ...**
>
> According to Aristotle, hands are the 'tool of tools'. In India, hands give blessings and symbolize strength and generosity. It is used to seal friendship. Placing your hands on someone or something can mean blessing or healing. Raising your hand can mean honesty. Hands on your heart can mean adoration or gratitude. Two hands coming together can symbolize peace and friendship.[198] Human hands are considered to be

> the highest form of evolution in primates, used as a tool, symbol or weapon.[199]

Hands allow you to experience dexterity and grasp things. Your hand is designed to receive, gather, collect and hold. The sense of grasping correlates with the sense of touch and is ruled by air. Air has subtle movement, and is associated with direction, velocity and change. Vata dosha is involved in the limbs. This dosha has five subdoshas. These are also referred to as the five vayus. Vyana vayu relates to the limbs and to all forms of circulation in the arms. It is an outwards and expanding movement, the fastest moving energy in the body.

It is critical to keep vata in mind in this chapter. It is vata imbalance that causes challenges with pain and is responsible for sleep disruption.

We will also explore the nervous and muscular systems in the hands, which, when impacted, severely affect your ability to grasp, and even impact future mobility, increase risk for heart disease and stroke.[200] Think of your grasp, or the strength of your grasp, as a powerful predisposing factor of more serious challenges.

How Pain Affects Your Sleep Quality

Areas in your brain which recognize pain signals also regulate sleep. Persistent pain causes lack of sleep or impacts its quality and, in turn, that poor sleep prevents chronic inflammation from shutting off. Recently, there has been more interest and research in the bidirectional aspect of sleep and pain.[201]

Symptoms of conditions like fibromyalgia include fatigue, impaired sleep and cognitive difficulties, but the main result of the disease is widespread chronic pain.

How Does the Ability to Grasp Impact Sleep?

Dhruv was in his early fifties and was facing great difficulties in grasping or holding something. This was unusual. He had been an avid golfer for decades and had recently been diagnosed with nerve damage, or tendonitis in his wrist, and had developed the first signs of rheumatoid arthritis, causing substantial inflammation in his hands and the joints of his arms. He was finding it difficult to grasp and hold anything, and what was impacting him the most was that he was finding it harder and harder to hold his golf club. I asked him, 'How is your sleep? Do you find pain impacting your sleep?'

Dhruv replied, 'I ignore it. Pain does bother me. I take a painkiller when it is bad.'

When there is inflammation in the muscles and joints, sleep is crucial since it heals soft tissues and muscles, and allows any scar tissue to form. When sleep is restricted, having higher than optimal protein can be supportive to the body.[202] But when scar tissues form, they can trap areas of soft tissues, causing shortening of muscles and tendons to get inflamed as tendonitis. It can also trap the nerves within, causing nerve impingement in the hands, leading to numbness, pain and shock. Like any golfer, Dhruv could not think of giving up golf. We settled on a six-week break from golf to give his system time for the inflammation to shut down.

I asked him, 'What do you think prevents you from experiencing deep sleep? Do you struggle with any pain in your hands through the night?'

He replied, 'I used to sleep on my abdomen, with my arms buried under me. But then I found I developed pain and numbness there a few hours later.' He was open to making drastic changes in his diet and lifestyle right away.

Understanding the Sense of Grasp

Dhruv had gradually developed loss of strength in his hands and the predisposing factors were repetitive usage from golf combined with an inflammatory diet. He was eating a diet which was high in boxed muesli, milk and fast food. Many nights a week, he was out binge drinking, relying on caffeine the next day. His blood sugar was all over the place.

He was not eating enough protein and his diet was quite low in omega-3. He had no idea that magnesium was important for hundreds of functions in the body.[203] I explained to him how necessary magnesium was in the transmission of signals within the nervous system. He was also eating a lot of Chinese food. I told him about glutamates in Chinese foods, and how they could produce inflammatory cytokines and result in chronic inflammation.[204]

Can Solving the Vata Puzzle Be the Answer to Pain and Sleep Problems?

Joint pains in the hands begin with excess vata in the whole body. The imbalance begins with weak agni and vata-aggravating practices. This can occur due to eating cold and dry foods. As vata increases, agni becomes even more weak. The weak agni then causes accumulation of ama, or metabolic toxins. This begins within the digestive tract.

The joints are gathering spaces of vata dosha. Ama is sticky. It shares qualities with kapha, which is responsible for cushioning the joint. There is agni within cells too. If agni is weak in any of the tissues, excess vata and ama penetrate, and start to dry the joints of the hand. Over time, the impact becomes severe.

One way to identify vata in the joints is if the joints feel cold, or if they often make popping and cracking sounds. Remember that when vata is aggravated, it brings with it all kinds of sleep challenges. This includes pain as well.

To soothe vata in the joints, you must focus on calming vata overall, as mentioned in the chapter on sound and the adrenals. Locally, you can add warming and soothing herbal oils. Dhanwantaram, mahanarayana tailam, murivenna, or warm sesame oil, are wonderful for this. Massage your hands after you have applied warm sesame oil to the whole body to calm vata dosha. Maintaining a circadian rhythm that is in harmony with the earth's diurnal rhythm is critical to calming vata dosha. It is also key that the foods you eat are soft, warm and cooked, and not cold or dry. It is helpful to first eliminate the aggravating factors such as caffeine. Without eliminating them, other protocols may not be as effective.

33

Hands, Muscles and Nerves

Before you can grasp something, you must reach out for it, which involves controlling your torso and head, as well as moving your eyes. Have you ever thought about how evolved a function grasping is? It is an extremely fascinating sense organ. The ability to grasp makes the hand an amazingly versatile tool, allowing you to manipulate the smallest of objects.

Your thumb allows you to perform so many functions. Try folding your thumb and trying to grasp something—it is nearly impossible. Your hands are also used to touch and feel things. Your hands consist of four different nerve endings that make your fingers so sensitive and allow them to grasp.

Skeletal and Muscular Structure of Hands

What can really help the health of your hands, and support you in the prevention of inflammation and poor grasp, is structural movement and exercise developed for healthy blood circulation. Your hand involves the arrangement of twenty-seven small bones. Eight carpal bones make up your wrist and these are neatly arranged into two rows. Fine long metacarpal bones make up your palm. They connect the wrist to your fingers. Each of your fingers contain three phalanges, except for your thumb, which contains only two.

Thirty-five powerful muscles move your hands. Fifteen are in your forearm and the rest in your hands. This arrangement is what gives your hand such strength and dexterity. Close to your wrist, the muscles are stronger, forming slender cords called tendons. These run all along your palm and the back of your hands right up to the joints in your fingers. When the muscles in your palms and forearms contract, your fingers close, allowing you to grasp. When the muscles on the back of your forearms contract, the fingers open. There are twenty muscles just within your hands that are arranged in a way such that your fingers and hands can make these precise movements such as grasping.

The Nervous System and Pain

Your nervous system is the body's internal electrochemical network involved in communication. The brain, spinal cord and nerves comprise your nervous system. Your brain and spine make up your central nervous system, which is the main controlling and coordinating centre.

Billions of neurons, grouped together as nerves, make up the peripheral nervous system, which connects your brain and spinal cord to your arms and hands. They transmit signals from the brain and spinal cord to your hands, allowing delicate and sophisticated movements. This part of your nervous system is called the somatic or voluntary peripheral nervous system, which involves nerves that serve your limbs, including your hands. It includes muscle, skeletal and exterior sense organs which work like receptors for your brain, receiving valuable information.

Without optimal functioning of the nervous system, you will not be able to use your hands in all the possible ways and you will lack dexterity. Remember that it is vata dosha that is responsible for the functioning of your nervous system and your hands! Taking a pause during the day, during which time you lie down on the ground and listen to a guided meditation, is a practice that is always supportive to calming vata dosha.

The peripheral nervous system also includes the autonomic nervous system and the enteric nervous system within your gut. The autonomic nervous system involves your sympathetic and parasympathetic nervous system, which I have discussed in detail in several places in this book. Every area of the nervous system undergoes sleep-stage dependant or circadian changes during sleep. One study described the different areas of the nervous system and the connection to sleep perfectly:

> The autonomic nervous system (ANS) controls vital bodily functions such as cardiovascular and respiratory regulation that are strongly influenced by sleep. Sleep induces profound changes in the function of the ANS and components of the ANS are involved in circadian rhythm and stimulation of melatonin. Physiological differences between wakefulness, non-rapid eye movement (NREM) sleep, and rapid eye movement (REM) or paradoxical sleep are mediated through alteration of the sympathetic and parasympathetic nervous systems as well as diminution and inhibition of the somatic sensory and motor nervous systems. NREM sleep is generally characterised by parasympathetic dominance, slow rolling eye movements, decreased muscle tone,

heart rate, breathing, blood pressure, metabolic rate, and temperature, while REM sleep contrasts by both tonic and phasic sympathetic enhancement, increased blood pressure, heart rate, metabolism, and rapid eye movements. Changes in gastrointestinal track and ENS are largely guided by circadian influences; however, some sleep-dependent modulations and ANS influence are at play.[205]

When it comes to your nervous system, oxygenation is key. Having a shallow breath can cause inflammation to the hands or arms.

If your blood sugar management is poor, then you may face insulin resistance or have less than optimal blood sugar patterns. Both low blood sugar and insulin resistance impact how much glucose reaches your brain. Brain health and blood sugar may very well be a bidirectional axis.

34

Pain and Sleep

What Is Chronic Inflammation?

Acute inflammation is when you fall and get hurt, and your immune system responds to protect you by causing heat, redness, swelling or pain. Eventually, all these subside and the inflammation shuts off. In chronic inflammation, where an area of your body remains in a continual state of inflammation, it confuses your immune system. Your immune system reacts with swelling or pain, and if you repeatedly do something which causes it to launch an attack, then you stay in a state of chronic inflammation, where it does not shut off, impacting your nerves and muscles.

There are many things that cause a negative impact to your immune system. Eating foods that are inflammatory, hard to digest or unsuitable to your body constitution in the form of starches, processed foods, desserts and alcohol can keep your body in a state of inflammation. You can cause muscle damage or strain in a state of inflammation. Alcohol is a major reason for staying in a state of inflammation, and so is smoking.[206]

Painkillers are another source. Three days of taking them becomes ten. A week becomes a month, until eventually you start relying on medicines to get through the day.[207] These medications are also triggers of vata aggravation and weaken agni.

Studies have shown that NSAID drugs like Ibuprofen lead to mucosal damages, including erosions and ulceration.[208] They destroy mucosa over time and make your epithelium permeable, leading to inflammation.

When it comes to your hands and wrists, in conditions like fibromyalgia, tendonitis or arthritis, perpetuating inflammation can cause damage to nerves. Damaged tissues release chemicals that communicate with nerves. This pain information travels to the spinal cord and brain. The brain recognizes pain, but the areas of the brain that recognize pain also control sleep. While Western research is looking further into the research between pain and sleep,[209] in Ayurveda, pain and poor sleep are said to be caused by excess vata.

Another point to note is that some medications, especially painkillers, prescribed for conditions that impact your hands, wrists and arms like fibromyalgia, arthritis and tendonitis, can increase overall inflammation and negatively impact sleep.

The Usual Suspects of Inflammation

1. The first immune culprit is localized strain. Pushing your body beyond its limit is vata aggravating.
2. Excessive sugar can be a major immune culprit.[210] Sugar in the form of a high carbohydrate diet, excessive starches, sweets and alcohol suppress white blood cells and their response.

3. Nutrient deficiencies are another cause.[211] Your immune system requires multiple nutrients for optimal function. Poor agni that accompanies high vata can prevent the absorption of nutrients, even in a good diet.
4. In today's world, the biggest immune culprit is toxic exposure.[212]
5. Without controlling stress, nothing else can be effective. High stress raises cortisol and increases inflammation. Inflammation can also be a result of excess pitta. Vata stokes the fire of pitta. Excess heat from pitta can increase dryness, in turn, aggravating vata. It helps to calm both with deep relaxation activities.
6. Antibiotics and painkillers are a big threat. Antibiotics impact your microbiome and make you immune sensitive, and painkillers damage the mucosa, stressing your immune system.[213] Medication is another vata-aggravating trigger.
7. Work on strengthening agni so that you can move beyond food allergies. Instead of accumulation of ama from weak agni, your body can nourish your tissues.

How You Can Achieve a Balanced Immune System

While there are many immune culprits, there are also several ways to support immune function and lower inflammation. These can be wonderful resources on your journey of lowering chronic inflammation.

1. An anti-inflammatory diet is step one. The antioxidants in colourful plant foods have potent powers to fight any free radical damage within your body.[214]
2. Try a short healing phase where you reduce glutamates. These are compounds found in MSG, yeast, soy sauce, parmesan,

sauerkraut, gelatine, peas, corn and tomatoes. Remove these for a trial period of two to four weeks and observe how you feel. These are best kept away. Nightshades like tomatoes, potatoes and peppers have benzoic acid, which is a toxin that causes joint pain. In the event of pain, it is best to remove them.

3. Spices like ginger, cinnamon, garlic, turmeric, nutmeg, clove, cardamom, rosemary and thyme fire agni and decrease inflammation, preserving the brain's fatty acid integrity and helping to lower pain.[215] Remember to simmer the spices in fat to improve digestibility of food.
4. Vitamins A, C, D, E, B2, B6 and B12, folic acid, iron and selenium are important for the immune system.[216] The best way to include all the nutrients that you need is through a varied and colourful diet.
5. Reduce or eliminate alcohol. It aggravates vata and pitta.
6. Improve oxygen flow. Get enough exercise, include inversions from yoga if you do not have high blood pressure, stand on one leg and go for long walks.
7. Meditation is magical! It has been proven to lower brain inflammation, help nerve recovery and improve resilience.[217]
8. Zinc is an immune wonder.[218] Get it from pumpkin seeds, squash seeds, sunflower seeds, seafood, oysters, liver, turkey, crab, herring, organ meats, mushrooms, soybeans, eggs, rice, sesame seeds and legumes.
9. Omega-3 is not optional.[219] You can get ALA from greens, flax, chia, hemp, ghee and walnuts. You need the EPA and DHA from fatty fish, algae or full-fat ghee.
10. Love, learn, laugh. Love increases oxytocin and reduces anxiety, supporting pain and inflammation reduction.[220] Learning new things or doing puzzles are known to improve neurogenesis, or the production of new nerve cells, helping

to lower brain inflammation and reduce pain.[221] Laughing reduces stress and increases neurotransmitters like beta-endorphins, which are your body's natural painkillers.

Supporting Recovery from Pain to Improve Sleep

When it comes to pain and sleep, as is evident by now, it can be a delicate situation of the chicken or the egg. Which came first? Where do you begin? Poor sleep can be very disruptive to pain, but it's much harder to force sleep than it is to work on your system and reduce pain. Focus on strengthening agni and pacifying vata.

Your nervous and immune systems respond to both fear and love. It is common to stay in fear, panicking over the helplessness of your situation and being unable to move away from that towards hope and future resolution. High vata can make you more anxious and fearful. But also know that these systems respond to love as well. Chronic and persistent pain is a sensory and emotional response. Love produces oxytocin and it is remarkable for lowering inflammation. Adverse childhood experiences are powerful triggers and mediators in inflammation. If you have been through situations like those, it would be useful to explore how that trauma can be reduced with tools like therapy and meditation.

What were those situations that caused you to feel fear or anxiety? When did you face them? Are you dealing with such a situation today, and if so, what can you do about it? Keep a journal and really get to the root of your inflammation.

35

Therapies for Your Sense of Grasping

Therapies and nutrients in this chapter are specific to supporting the sense of grasping, and quelling inflammation and pain. Some of these are part of the ten-sense protocol.

Replenish Micronutrients for the Nerves and Pain

If your problem lies with inflammation in your arms and hands, these nutrients may be beneficial for you.

Turmeric helps heal the mucous membranes, get your bile flowing, mobilizes movement of toxic stagnation and supports lymphatic movement to release toxins. It is part of the highly anti-inflammatory ginger family. It has been used in Eastern wisdom for centuries. It also boosts BDNF, and is a powerful tool against anxiety and for sleep. Be cautious about turmeric supplements. Always check with a health practitioner before adding turmeric as it interacts with several drugs. It is always better to begin using spices simmered in ghee, strengthening agni and calming vata, which are more powerful than using turmeric as a pill or shot.

Vitamin A is an immune powerhouse and its deficiency is associated with inflammatory conditions. Deficiency can cause a breakdown of the mucosa. It can also lead to thymus atrophy and strain your immune system. Vitamin A is found in foods like egg yolks, liver, whole milk, spinach, carrots, yellow or dark-green vegetables, cod liver oil, fermented cod liver oil, mint, turnip greens, orange fruits, vegetables, squash, mangoes, dandelion, kale, tuna, mackerel and fish liver oils.

Sadhana or Therapies

Think of adding a dedicated sadhana for nurturing each of your senses and your body will undergo dramatic changes.

Chinese Medicine Balls

Try using Tibetan stress balls. As I have mentioned earlier, they improve dexterity and calm your sense of sleep. Hold two balls in your hands and keep rotating them, trying to change their position while they still touch each other. Keep moving them around in different ways, being aware of the tension in your hands reducing.

Play with Clay

Playing with clay is a great way to build strength in your hands. Long ago, I asked a young girl who was recuperating from surgery of her wrist to knead dough. Go back to feeling like a child, create something with your hands and allow the coolness of the clay to work its therapeutic magic on you. Squish it into a ball, roll it around, make long snakes, wrap them around each other and roll them around. It would even be fun to join a pottery class, where you can have access to a potter's wheel.

Sense Withdrawal to Soothe Grasp

What better way to restrain your sense of grasp than to practice mudras? Mudras may have symbolic value in some religions, but there is deep, ancient wisdom behind practising them. They are a rich part of the yoga tradition and are powerful tools to restrain or rest your sense of grasp. Think of mudras as hand positions that can channelize your energy in specific ways and with specific intentions.

Vyana mudra calms down vyana vayu. Here are the simple steps to practice vyana mudra:

1. Start with the apana mudra: Touch the tips of the ring and middle fingers to the tip of the thumb, while keeping the index and little finger extended.
2. Now move the tip of the index finger to the crease at the base of the thumb, keeping palms facing up and little extended.
3. Holding this in meditation, make sure that your palms are facing up to the ceiling while you rest your hands on your thighs.
4. The touch should be subtle as you become sensitive to your nerves.

How Dhruv Resolved His Sleep by Understanding His Pain

Dhruv focused on removing the triggers of imbalance in his life. He understood that this was more powerful than any protocol. He focused on eating wholesome, nourishing, warm and moist foods at home. Every morning and evening, he spent five minutes holding vyana mudra to help calm vata dosha. He kept a journal every day to release all that he could not express to anyone and noticed how he started to feel more stable. He included abhyanga with sesame oil or a medicated oil four or five days a week. As vata calmed down, his pain disappeared. To help him sleep deeply, he also started to lie on his back while covering his ears and head with a cap. With time, he was healed and felt like a new person altogether.

PART 11

The Tenth Sense: Speech

36

Speech, the Thyroid Gland and Resilience

You may be wondering why the thyroid gland features in a chapter about speech. The thyroid gland is a butterfly-shaped gland that sits within your throat, between the collarbones. It controls a tremendous number of functions, and is intricately connected to both sleep and speech. If your thyroid gland does not produce enough hormone, one symptom is a hoarse voice or impacted speech. If the thyroid gland is enlarged, one of the concerns is frequent coughing and lots of challenges with speech. Deficiency of the thyroid hormone may be at the root of impaired speech. The sense of speech or expression correlates with the sense of sound and is ruled by ether. Ether is associated with communication, self-expression and connection.

Research has found that thyroid deficiency is at the root of dryness in the larynx and the feeling of a lump in the throat. Fundamental frequency in speech is the speed at which vocal cords vibrate, and correlates with the pitch of your voice. Thyroid deficiency impacts this fundamental frequency, altering your voice.[222]

The Role of the Butterfly Gland

The thyroid gland is an endocrine gland, a chemical messenger. Your thyroid is located in front of your trachea, at the base of your throat. It is a small gland with a powerful job. It secretes hormones which have a massive impact on overall health and metabolism.

Your thyroid gland regulates your body temperature, controls metabolism, and regulates appetite, libido, sleep and psychological behaviours. Thyroid malfunction or thyroid hormone deficiency can lead to symptoms such as fatigue, inability to exercise, a swollen thyroid gland, poor metabolism, joint pains, weight gain, hair fall, dry skin, depression, anxiety, irritability, allergies, hives, oedema, feeling too hot or too cold, slow heart rate, constipation, hormonal imbalance, menstrual irregularities, snoring and poor sleep quality. An overactive thyroid, on the other hand, can cause symptoms such as weight loss, excessive appetite, irritability, increased heart rate, inability to wind down, nervousness, palpitations and insomnia.

How Your Sense of Speech Impacts Your Sleep

Rania evoked my empathy because she had been struggling with terrible sleep for months and it was starting to impact every area of her life. Sometimes, she resisted speaking what was on her mind for a variety of reasons, and sometimes she burst out in fury, torn by anger and sadness at the same time. She was diagnosed with hypothyroidism a few years ago. Try as she might, with medication and a variety of health approaches, she struggled to feel energized through the day and had poor sleep at night. She either woke up tired even after nine to ten hours of sleep or, if she failed to sleep at the right time, she struggled to fall asleep or stay asleep.

She felt many of life's choices were thrust on her. She could not afford to take time off to recover if she fell sick. She struggled working two jobs. She felt frustrated when her friends suggested she take a vacation because she felt that they did not understand her situation. She just could not afford one.

I asked her, 'Do you wake up tired every single day?'

She replied, 'Almost. There are days I wake up refreshed, provided I have had an uninterrupted nine to ten hours of sleep, but it is quite rare.'

She said that she struggled with people asking her if she had a sore throat, but, over time, her voice had become hoarse. Eventually, she felt it was better to make up stories simply because she was tired of receiving loose advice, recommendations that did not work and a general lack of understanding.

She told me that she had a lot of stress, probably way more than what was healthy, and she had numbed herself to it.

I asked her, 'What do you think prevents you from having deep sleep? Can you pinpoint what is the biggest problem with sleep?'

She replied, 'In the last few months, I have definite issues with finding comfort in my bedroom. When my husband says it is cold and wants a blanket, I am sweating and cannot fall asleep. When he feels hot, I feel cold and I am shivering, and there is such discomfort through my body that sleep feels uncomfortable to me.'

Rania was being totally honest with me and she mentioned that this was the first time she could really open with anyone. I asked her about what she did to cope with stress and whether she was trying to incorporate practices that might improve her resilience. She felt she did not have time.

I asked her if she had a meditation practice. She did not. Meditation and yoga can be powerful tools to help thyroid function since the source of all endocrine function is at the brain.[223]

Understanding Your Sense of Speech

The mouth is the sense organ which allows you to experience speech. It allows you to share what is on your mind and can be a voice into your soul. Your mouth represents communication, your ability or inability to speak what is on your mind, and allows you to interact with the world.

Speech refers to communication that is verbal. Have you ever experienced a time in your life when you found someone suppressing your speech or when you could not control yourself and words burst out? Rania spoke about her mother, who would glare at her and silence her multiple times because she never liked any form of conflict. Can you visualize a wine bottle, sealed with a cork and left for ages to ferment? At some point, it will explode, the wine bursting out. This is what was happening to Rania. Speech is a powerful way through which you can express yourself and it is an area which requires immense balance. The world cannot read your emotions and thoughts, and speech allows you to overcome this barrier.

Is There a Magical Tip to Help the Brain and Speech?

Your brain is such a fascinating part of your body. If you recall, I had talked about the right and left hemispheres of the cerebrum being separated by a long fissure known as the corpus callosum. The cerebrum is filled with folds that serve to increase your brain's surface area. These folds divide your cerebrum into four lobes. The anterior frontal lobe make speech possible. This is the left side of your cerebrum. Your cerebrum is also considered the newest part of the brain, and therefore responsible for higher functions such as speech, which other species cannot do.

What could help this part of your brain? Research has found a connection between those who have been practising meditation for a long time and the thickness of the corpus callosum. This suggests that meditation can improve the communication in the cerebrum and promote improved speech.[224] This can support improved resilience, calmness, balance and the ability to speak from a space of truth which is also free of aggression.

Speech quality reflects resilience and has roots in deeper systems of biology. Frequent angry speech can indicate systemic inflammation. This connection has been spoken about in Traditional Chinese Medicine and Ayurveda, and some research into it has furthered this understanding.[225]

A Healing Routine for Speech

The voice and speech are connections to the outside world. There is so much you can do to support your speech.

1. Stop overworking or misusing your voice. Nurture your sense of speech by reducing shouting and giving periods of rest to your voice. If your voice ever feels hoarse, strained or sore, soothe your throat with healing foods such as aloe vera juice.
2. While kapha dosha is related to the throat, all the doshas play a role in thyroid health. Excess vata dosha increases dryness in the body. Vata aggravation can impact the throat and speech. Increased vata also imbalances the nervous system and adrenal

function. These play an integral role in thyroid health and sleep. High vata also imbalances agni and weak agni is very much interconnected with thyroid issues. Dry throat is a vata symptom and may require cutting out dry foods, favouring warm, moist, cooked foods.
3. Drink enough fluids to keep your throat hydrated. Vocal cords keep vibrating and can feel strained from frequent speech. Having enough fluids maintains the water balance and lubricates your throat. Caffeine and alcohol can dehydrate your throat further. Consume warm beverages through the day. Avoid drinking beverages with your meals as it can dilute digestive strength.
4. Do not clear your throat too many times in a day. It is almost like bashing your vocal cords against each other. If you feel like clearing your throat, try sipping some fluid instead.
5. Maintaining silence or mouna is an ancient practice aimed at bringing about balanced speech. Observing a day of silence will help calm vata as well. Excess speech imbalances vata dosha and a high vata symptom is excess speech.
6. Stop smoking as it can hurt your voice. Active and passive smoke can destroy vocal cords and leave your throat constantly tired.
7. Humidifier helps sleep. Always remember that moisture is excellent for your voice and speech.

37

The Miracle Gland: The Thyroid

Your thyroid is located just in front of your trachea, at the base of your throat. This gland regulates your body temperature, controls metabolism, regulates appetite, libido, sleep and psychology. Some features of the gland to keep in mind are:

1. The brain is critically important to thyroid function. The pituitary gland is the master gland within your brain. It is just the size of a pea and sits within the cranial bone. The anterior pituitary secretes TSH, or thyroid stimulating hormone (TSH), which promotes production of the hormone and release from your thyroid gland. In response to TSH, the thyroid gland releases T4 and a little T3. T4 is the inactive form of thyroid hormone and gets converted to the active form of T3 in the gut, liver, muscles and kidneys.[226]
2. Trauma to your head and autoimmunity can impact thyroid function right at the source within your brain.
3. T3 and T4 play a role in the brain's health. If your thyroid is not fully functional, then it can also show up as depression, anxiety, poor sleep or irritability. Hypothyroidism can correlate to mood disruption and possible low serotonin, leading to

alteration in the HPT axis. If you struggle with mental health challenges and poor sleep, managing thyroid dysfunction optimally is critical. Thyroid, adrenal health and sleep are intricately connected.[227]

4. Your hypothalamus is connected to your pituitary gland. It stimulates the gland to release hormones. It can detect high or low levels of an organ's hormones and then send hormonal or electrical signals to the pituitary gland to either release or stop hormone production. If temperature is too low, the hypothalamus makes the body generate and maintain heat. If current body temperature is too high, heat is given off or sweat is produced to cool the skin.[228] It also releases TRH, or thyrotropin releasing hormone, and stimulates the pituitary to release TSH.

5. TSH then triggers the thyroid gland to release thyroid hormones. All this happens through communication within the HPT axis. T4 is secreted after the release of TSH, which requires an amino acid called tyrosine and adequate iodine. For optimal thyroid function, you need the right amount of iodine, selenium, zinc, ferritin and stomach acid, great liver function and a healthy brain.

6. If your immune system tags a specific food like gluten with an antibody, deciding that it is a pathogen, it can look like other tissue in the body, like your thyroid. This is called molecular mimicry. It then attacks the thyroid gland. In fact, you train it to attack the gland. Each time you eat gluten again, it attacks similar molecules. Try a short four-week elimination phase and observe how your body responds. Listen to your own body.

7. Digestive health plays a major role in thyroid function.[229] Thyroid dysfunction always begins at the intersection between

genetics, poor gut health and pathogenic microbiome.[230] Those with hypothyroidism struggle with substantially poor levels of bile flow, impacting fat digestion and detoxification.[231] Low iron levels can impact thyroid health.[232] If you have low iron, you can experience chronic fatigue, anxiety or restless legs syndrome. These impact sleep.

8. Nutrient deficiencies play a major role in both the development of thyroid challenges, as well as the ability to manage any thyroid dysfunction. B vitamins play a very important role in all health.[233] They are involved in acetylcholine production, which is key to the parasympathetic nervous system, and therefore sleep.[234] Unsupervised low carb diets can deplete several vitamins. Look at sources of natural salt instead, such as celery, sea vegetables in moderation, seafood and good sea salt.

9. When it comes to your thyroid health, blood sugar and adrenal balance play a role as well. Go back to the section on steps for adrenal recovery and make sure that you have dealt with your stress before digging deeper into thyroid issues. Stress is key to thyroid health.[235]

How Are Your Thyroid and Adrenals Connected to Your Sleep?

Your adrenal glands are responsible for your energy and for how you sleep. While the stress hormone is produced in the outer shell of your adrenal gland, the inner medulla produces adrenaline and this also gets overproduced in high stress. This region is also the space where the amino acid tyrosine gets converted to adrenaline.[236] Tyrosine is critical to thyroid function as well.[237] If there is excessive stress and tyrosine is converted to adrenaline, then it impacts thyroid function.

Low thyroid also causes dips in your energy. Thyroid dysfunction, poor sleep and adrenal issues are deeply connected. Therefore, the solution requires looking at all three.[238] The thyroid also plays a role in your circadian rhythm. Thyroid dysfunction can reduce slow wave sleep.[239] Remember that adrenal dysfunction is associated with vata aggravation.

As you can see, your thyroid gland has many connections to the quality of your sleep. There is also a connection between your thyroid and your circadian rhythm. Research has shown that those working at times which upset the circadian rhythm have a higher risk of developing thyroid dysfunction.[240]

Hashimoto's disease, or autoimmune thyroid dysfunction, is becoming increasingly common today, leading to immense challenges to overall health, temperature regulation and sleep. Sleep disorders left unattended can cause thyroid dysfunction.[241]

A sluggish thyroid and thyroid hormone deficiency can make you feel fatigued even after excessive sleep. The drop in metabolism caused by low thyroid hormones is what makes your body feel dull, sluggish and tired. Hypothyroid could also be a factor impacting slow wave sleep. Slow wave sleep makes you feel refreshed after deep sleep. Without this stage of deep sleep, no amount of sleep can be healing. Taking afternoon naps can even make it worse.

Your hypothalamus, which is a major player in thyroid health, is also your body's thermostat. When you have thyroid challenges, this thermostat behaves as if it's broken. It can cause you to have night sweats and wake up soaking in your own sweat sometimes. Then, it can make you feel excessively cold, irrespective of all attempts to keep yourself warm. Hypothyroid also causes a drop in core body temperature as a result of slow metabolism.

RLS causes poor sleep quality and one of the causes of this is TSH levels.[242] Magnesium deficiency can also be a factor. Calming vata dosha plays an integral role here.

Thyroid imbalance can cause imbalance in sex hormones like oestrogen. Low thyroid hormones can cause oestrogen levels to drop.[243] Menopausal women with low oestrogen and progesterone can suffer from insomnia.[244] Low oestrogen levels can cause hot flashes, abrupt interruptions to sleep and difficulty falling back asleep. Low progesterone can cause sleep anxiety.

Hyperthyroidism, on the other hand, can cause insomnia due to palpitations, racing heart and anxiety. Those with adrenal dysfunction also struggle to wind down and sleep. Supporting adrenal health and recovery can be supportive to promoting sleep if your thyroid is underactive or overactive.

As you can see, the body is beautifully interlinked. I would like you to reframe your mindset now. If you have been thinking that every system in your body is broken, I would like you to change this perspective today. Instead, what if you think *every system in your body is beautifully interconnected*, and therefore, *whatever you do to positively influence one system today can be powerful in influencing many other systems as well*, helping you restore overall balance?

Thyroid, Temperature and Sleep

Do you feel hot or cold when no one else in the room does?

In a normal human body, thyroid hormones increase energy, regulate body temperature, appetite, fat build-up, sleep and weight. They work with your nervous system to maintain this temperature. Thyroid hormones decide how much ATP, or the energy molecule, will be created. The more ATP you produce, the more efficient you will be in generating heat. If you produce too much, you will sweat. Those with thyroid underactivity will produce much less heat. Most heat is created within brown fat, which is important for adjusting to cold weather.[245]

It has been found that the thyroid hormone is a key player in vascular regulation of body temperature. The findings of this interesting study can add to what is already known about temperature oversensitivity experienced by patients with thyroid disorders. In the long run, the discovery might possibly lead to treatments that correct dysfunctional vascular regulation.[246]

Basal body temperature should normally be around 36.5–36.7 degrees Celsius. Consistently having lower temperature is indicative of hypothyroidism and having higher temperatures can be indicative of hyperthyroidism. Oral body temperature is normally 37.1–37.3 degrees Celsius. If you struggle with temperature fluctuations and thyroid dysfunction, which impact your sleep, it will be useful to monitor this temperature and support yourself in ways that promote sleep. Good sleep requires a cooler core body temperature. If you find yourself having consistently elevated temperature, a cool water soak can restore some homeostasis. This can also be a result of high pitta. You can also cope better with movement and exercise. If you find yourself feeling cold all the time, it can be high vata or kapha. We are all unique and need different tools at different times. Being mindful will help us to choose the right one. When in doubt, a simple abhyanga, with warm oil before a bath, helps to support us in our own ability to manage temperature. Always remind yourself that agni plays a role in our ability to regulate temperature.

Thyroid function and adrenal health both play a role in temperature regulation. The season, time of day, circadian alignment, diet, sex hormones and sleep quality can all play a role as well.

Supporting Thyroid Recovery to Improve Sleep

Supporting thyroid health begins with digestion, gut health, microbial diversity, liver health, adrenal function and hormone balance.

The first thing to understand is that there is no perfect diet. People may have told you to eat only for two hours in a day or to stick to a vegan or paleo diet. Such advice need not work on everyone. You truly are unique. Discover what is best for you and stick to it.

Healing Routine for Thyroid Health and Better Sleep

When it comes to addressing thyroid health, remember to move step by step and be consistent with each step.

1. Gluten is thought to be a problem. Staying away for a short while and seeing how your body responds can be insightful. Once you strengthen your agni, you may introduce it again. It may work for some and may not for others. If there is excess kapha, then wheat can be too heavy. Those with thyroid challenges have a tendency to have low stomach acid. Make sure you support this with some ginger to build agni. You do not need to be on a low-carb diet, but consider a diet that is low in sugar and starch. Include plenty of wholesome and complex carbohydrates, including non-starchy vegetables, jowar, bajra, ragi, amaranth, quinoa, millet, buckwheat, sweet potatoes, tapioca and rice. Removing gluten to allow your gut to recover from inflammation helps promote its repair and improves metabolism. Make sure that you have proteins

which are easy to digest and supportive to healing until your digestion has improved. In deep thyroid dysfunction, proteins like beans can be very challenging on digestion until agni is stronger. If you eat animal protein, fish can be a wonderful option, as is collagen powder. If you follow a plant-based diet, stay with lighter proteins like soaked seeds and lighter lentils. Another option is to complement a great diet with high-quality organic pea protein.

2. Tyrosine is found in foods like avocado, almonds, spinach, tuna, duck, turkey, beef, salmon and leafy greens. You can ensure a complete amino acid profile simply by eating balanced meals that include carbohydrates, proteins and fats. You do not have to fear cruciferous vegetables like kale, cauliflower and cabbage unless you are consuming large amounts of them raw in smoothies. Eating a simple cooked cruciferous vegetable is liver supportive.

3. Check your iron levels. Iron is required in many areas of thyroid production.[247] Anything that you do to calm vata and strengthen agni is supportive.

4. Stress affects thyroid function as it can cause excessive production of reverse T3 instead of active T3.[248] Always remind yourself of how high vata impairs agni.

5. Vitamins help. B vitamins are required for thyroid health. B1 helps with fatigue, mood,[249] sleep and energy levels. B vitamins also help liver detoxification and improve metabolism, reducing stress on your body from the symptoms of thyroid dysfunction.

6. Exercise regularly. Movement and exercise are deeply beneficial to thyroid health and improving sleep. It improves secretion of thyroid hormones and receptivity.[250]

7. People with thyroid challenges have microbial imbalance with higher pathogenic bacteria, yeast overgrowth and parasites.[251] Having these pathogenic microbes in your intestine increases permeability and inflammation, making you predisposed to food allergies and autoimmune challenges. This can occur if you have had a lifetime of frequent antibiotics, high-sugar diets or a diet with little diversity. Weak agni is at the core of microbial attack, as is imbalance of kapha.
8. Since temperature can be a major factor with sleep, even more so with thyroid dysfunction, making sure that you set the right room temperature is important. The optimum temperature is considered to be between 16 to 21 degrees Celsius. Regular abhyanga, calming vata and strengthening agni are powerful tools to manage body temperature.
9. Support a healthy circadian cycle. Go to bed and wake up at set times. Thyroid function is intrinsically connected to circadian cycles. Darkness is supportive to deep sleep, healing and REM. Use an eye mask or make sure your room is dark.

38

Therapies for Your Sense of Speech

Use the Ancient Mystical Energy Encased in a Sound Structure

Speech connects the heart and the voice. A mantra is a mystical energy that is encased in a sound structure. With its repetition, you can tune into a higher state of consciousness, one that is supportive to entering a meditative state.

Sit somewhere where you can be comfortable. It is not important that you sit in any ideal posture. Just try to be comfortable and steady. Choose a mantra which you connect to, irrespective of religious connotation. If you do not connect to any, you can pick a positive and powerful affirmation which you would like to come true in your life. Repeat it aloud for a chosen number of times. As you keep chanting, you may find yourself reciting it softly and subtly, until it eventually becomes a whisper. This is a natural progression for chanting. It just means that you are moving towards a meditative state. This also allows for variety, which makes your mind feel that the practice is interesting. Keep your affirmation to yourself. Do not share it with everyone else.

Sit quietly for some time after you finish. Keep your eyes closed. Observe your mind and your thoughts.

Replenish Micronutrients for Your Thyroid

Even though the steps and supplements I present here are researched and designed to work well for most people with sleep challenges, remember to stay aware and observe your own body for feedback. Consider your diet, lifestyle, stressors, routine and symptoms. These are specific thyroid nutrients. Others which support thyroid are already listed in the ten-sense protocol as baseline supplements, including B-complex, omega-3, vitamin D and magnesium. Avoid adding something if you feel it is out of your scope to monitor or consult a skilled practitioner.

Thiamine or Vitamin B1

Thiamine is an integral part of many thyroid supplements. It acts as a co-enzyme to release energy from carbohydrates and fats. It is involved in the transmission of nerve signals. It forms collagen, which is critical to gut healing and recovery. It is also required for release of HCL by the stomach, and therefore connected to iron absorption and protein breakdown.

Selenium

Conversion of T4 to T3 is dependent on selenium.[252] Diets low in selenium can be a problem for thyroid function and can be a reason for developing autoimmune thyroid dysfunction or Hashimoto's disease. Selenium can reduce antibodies and improve energy levels.

Zinc

Zinc is a co-factor in your metabolic cycle. It is also very important for gut health, healing, conversion of T4 to T3 and the production of TSH.[253] Depletion can increase fungus and become a root cause for thyroid challenges.

Iron

Iron-deficiency symptoms can be similar to those of thyroid dysfunction. Low levels are often found in those with thyroid dysfunction. As those with thyroid challenges have a tendency for low stomach acid, it can impact the absorption and utilization of iron.

Sadhana or Therapies

Humming Your Way to Deep Sleep

The sound of humming within the brain is immensely tranquil and calming. It relieves stress. Humming is said to release cerebral tension as well. It releases anxiety and strengthens the throat. Since sound, speech, thyroid and the throat are all connected, humming is a great way to add a sadhana for your sense of speech. When you hum, you should feel a calming vibration in your mouth and your throat. Once you get into the practice, try different tones, scales and lengths. Make sure that your tongue stays down and doesn't move back towards your throat.

Journalling Your Way to Calmness

Journalling is a wonderful way to release words which you struggle to release through speech. First, get yourself a beautiful journal which attracts you with its creative design.

Journalling whatever comes in your mind the moment you wake up allows you to maintain clarity and great awareness through the day since it literally dumps what is bursting out of your mind before it comes out in negative ways through the day.

Ujjayi Pranayama

Ujjayi is a form of breathing that benefits the health of the throat specifically.

To practise it:

1. Sit comfortably. Partially close your glottis at the throat to form a soft sobbing sound at a uniform pitch.
2. Close your mouth and inhale through your nostrils smoothly.
3. Imagine there is a hole at your throat, between the two collarbones, and that you are drawing air through the hole at your throat. A smooth hiss should emanate from your throat, and you should be able to feel a sensation at your throat. This sound is sometimes referred to as ocean's breath.

It reduces all imbalances of the thyroid and stimulates pathways at the throat, which are healing and supportive to thyroid health. It should be avoided if there is excessively hyperactivity of the thyroid, but can be beneficial to thyroid health in general.

Sense Withdrawal to Soothe Your Speech

To restrain your sense of speech, practice mouna, or silence. Sit for a few minutes, perhaps after your brahmari, and listen to the sound of silence. Think of silence as that gap or pause between any two sounds. Practice mouna with austerity and mindfulness, so that it can lead you towards balanced speech. Make sure you remove yourself from all interactions, including your devices. When you practice, with time, you will not feel restless or irritable, but rather slip towards a state which is deeply peaceful and insightful.

How Rania Improved Her Sleep through Nurturing Her Sense of Speech

Rania started with journalling each morning so she could release all that was pent up within her.

She laid the foundations for a healthy thyroid by supporting agni and using castor oil packs for the liver. As she included abhyanga several times a week, she found her interaction with her space in terms of temperature regulation greatly improved. She avoided the air conditioner and started to open her windows. The combination of abhyanga and castor packs transformed her. She no longer feels unusually hot or cold. She spends ten minutes every night, sitting on her bed and humming quietly within herself. She has calmed down, her relationship has calmed down and her sleep quality improved. She now wakes up looking forward to the dawn of a new day.

Keep reading to uncover the ten-sense protocol, which is an overarching summary of the entire book, including the best ways to take care of every sense and building a protocol towards perfect sleep.

PART 12

The Ten-sense Protocol

The indriyas exist for our protection, and they are the bridge between our body and mind. Sound and speech are associated with the element of ether, which symbolizes space, communication and self-expression, and allows for connection. Touch and grasp are associated with the element of air, which symbolizes vata, subtle movement and change. Sight and locomotion are associated with the element of fire, which symbolizes light, perception and radiance, and allows movement. Taste and uro-reproduction are associated with the element of water, which symbolizes liquid and flowing motion and allows for life itself. Smell and detoxification are associated with the element of earth, symbolic of stability.

Through the ten-sense protocol, I'm going to take you through how to apply all that you've learned so far in a practical way, so that you can restore deep sleep. I've divided it into a four-week programme, where you can gradually immerse yourself deeper and deeper, step by step. Each week, you will be adding one practical application for each of the ten senses. Don't worry about having too much to do. The step are easy to follow and an example of a typical day is provided for each week. I'll also include information and methods to help you on your journey, such as ways to track the senses, how to discover your vulnerable sense, a basic supplement plan for the ten senses and so on. Don't worry if you cannot do everything I have suggested. Always appreciate yourself for whatever you can do. The more you can include, the sooner you will restore great sleep. I've built this protocol specifically with the thought of supporting every sense. But feel free to make changes based on what suits your body and lifestyle.

Look at the four-week approach as a chance to reset your life, where you will restore deep sleep, where sleep is the true medicine your mind and body need. You can be flexible with the approach and support only what needs to be supported. But I suggest that you first go through the four-week plan as I have laid it out so that you see the benefits and reach a space where you can then become flexible. It helps to write down how vulnerable you feel before you begin.

You've probably reached a point of poor sleep after a lifetime of stressors. You deserve the knowledge within this book to move towards a space of total recovery. Think of the next four weeks as a gift to yourself. It will transform your life, and allow you to work towards manifesting and achieving a greater purpose on this earth.

Before we head into the protocol, I want to add a quick section on the different root causes of sleep-onset insomnia versus sleep-maintenance insomnia.

Sleep-Onset Insomnia versus Sleep-Maintenance Insomnia

Sleep-onset insomnia refers to the inability to fall asleep. Sleep-maintenance insomnia refers to the inability to stay asleep. Perhaps you take a long time to fall asleep. Or maybe you fall asleep and then wake up at some point in the night, or even several times, and struggle to go back to sleep. Perhaps you struggle with both. If you struggle to stay asleep, and keep waking up and getting stressed, you probably lose out on several phases of deep sleep which are required for regeneration. The information below may be different from what traditional sleep science suggests. Keep an open mind and see what benefits you.

Root Causes of Sleep-Onset Insomnia

The inability to fall asleep is connected to almost every sense organ and all your systems. Here is a quick guide to help you discover which areas require your attention. You can go through all the chapters for more detailed information.

1. Stimulation through artificial light after sunset is a big reason. Vata is aggravated, thus affecting sleep.
2. A disrupted adrenal rhythm and elevated night-time cortisol disrupt sleep. Reduce sounds on all devices and avoid watching any TV or even reading a book that stimulates high adrenaline. Conduct a sound audit of your life. Supporting your sense of sound in several ways can help. Anything to calm vata is helpful.
3. Calm an overactive brain with aromatherapy.
4. Do you feel soothed and safe? Remember that oxytocin and cortisol share an antagonistic relationship. Abhyanga calms vata and lowers cortisol, boosting oxytocin.
5. Ultimately, your diet plays a major role. Focus on balancing meals while keeping agni strong.
6. Poor detoxification can raise night-time cortisol and adrenaline, making it difficult to fall asleep. Liver health is connected to your cortisol pattern. Supporting agni and calming vata will prevent constipation. Castor oil packs and abhyanga support detoxification.

7. If you struggle with falling asleep at specific times of the month, then the issue is related to hormone disharmony. That requires a deep look at your hormone health.
8. Lack of movement can cause sleep issues. Exercise raises core body temperature and subsequently lowers it, which can trigger asleep.
9. If you cannot fall asleep due to some pain, then addressing inflammation and calming vata are essential.

Root Causes of Sleep-Maintenance Insomnia

Issues with staying asleep intersect with the previous section. There are some differences, which include:

1. The body moves through many stages of sleep repeatedly through the night. If you wake up during lighter phases of sleep and there is light disturbance, it can easily trigger waking up. It is very important to minimize disturbances.
2. Cortisol has a natural rising rhythm sometime during sleep in preparation to wake you up. Waking up between 10 p.m.–2 a.m. is considered to be a sign of pitta imbalance. Waking up after 2 a.m. but before 4 a.m. is considered to be a sign of vata imbalance. While 4 a.m. to 6 a.m. is still vata time, it is also considered to be Brahma Muhurtham, an auspicious time to rise.
3. The glymph system detoxifies in the night. If you struggle with congestion, this issue is exacerbated at night-time as your brain attempts to detoxify. That can wake you up since you start breathing from your mouth due to the inability to breathe naturally through your nose. This can also cause

physical blockage and trigger sleep apnoea. Kapha imbalance is linked to weak agni.
4. Inadequate fluid intake during the day and too much fluid intake at night will hinder you from staying asleep. Keep electrolytes stable by consuming warm beverages through the day, though not near mealtime, and avoiding fluids after dinner.
5. Core body temperature is linked to both falling asleep and staying asleep. Regular abhyanga with warm sesame oil, a cool soak when your core body temperature is elevated and castor packs can help to manage temperature.
6. Restless legs can also be a reason for not staying asleep. Addressing pain and deficiencies, as well as stretching your large muscles regularly, can go a long way. Vata is linked to pain and restlessness.

Week 1

If you have already been making changes to your lifestyle, the four-week plan will allow you to bring in some structure to sustain and deepen your new habits. If you have not yet started, you can begin from scratch with this plan. Recommendations are made within frameworks for week. The main framework is a ten-step plan, which is simply one recommendation for every sense. Remember that the four-week plan is overarching and considers all ten senses.

The Ten-step Plan

1. Create a sacred sleep space.
2. Restrict the sounds in your life at night.
3. Create a space with soothing smells.
4. Start abhyanga to calm vata dosha.
5. Be grateful and chew your food well.
6. Add ginger as an appetizer to fire agni.
7. Try cold water therapy.
8. Walk barefoot.
9. Do shoulder rotations.
10. Improve your hydration.

1) Creating Your Sacred Sleep Space to Soothe Sight

Allow your heart and soul to speak to you in choosing a room colour. Blue and white are immensely soothing. Grey and muted pink are classics, they lend a charming vintage vibe. Moss green and dewy pink can feel relaxing, as do neutrals like taupe. It matters that you connect to the colours. The only thing to keep in mind is that if you have been struggling with sleep and your room has very bright colours, toning them down might be useful.

If you feel pain when you wake up or if you are not sleeping well, it may be time to change your mattress. I suggest going to a good store and trying out a few different varieties.

2) Restricting Sounds to Soothe the Sense of Sound

It is best to use an old-fashioned alarm clock and silence your phone altogether at night. I suggest having a fixed time to disconnect from all devices. For me, this is 5.00 p.m.

3) Create a Space with Soothing Smells

Breathe in the scent of your clean sheets and lavender oil. Take your time choosing the essential oil you like. See which ones touch your soul. Allow them to evoke memories that soothe your soul.

4) Abhyanga

Warm sesame oil abhyanga is calming to vata dosha and very helpful for sleep. If it is the height of summer in a hot location and you feel overheated, try using chemparuthyadi tailam. You can safely practise abhyanga for your body every day. Ideally, it is great if done in the morning, before a bath. But if you find yourself struggling with energy during the day, keep this for early evening, before dinner. It is wonderful to help you sleep.

5) Chewing to Soothe Taste

Chewing is a conscious practice. Its power is not used as it should be. Chew until your food is mush. Go back to all that supports healthy agni, such as eating three meals a day, no snacking, drinking warm water, not having fluids with meals and staying calm.

6) Ginger Appetizer

Ginger in moderation helps all doshas and may need to be introduced in small amounts if you have high pitta. Consuming a quarter teaspoon of ginger with a few drops of lime and a pinch of salt is powerful. If you feel excess heat or burning from the appetizer, consume less.

7) Cold Water Therapy to Support Uro Reproduction

Soak in a tub of cool water for ten minutes. Try this only once. If your body feels more equitable in temperature modulation, you don't need to do it again. Overdoing it will unbalance the body. After doing this once this week, switch to abhyanga and warm baths as often as possible.

8) Barefoot Walking

A wonderful way of moving lymph is with a long barefoot walk. It connects you to the earth, and is rooting and grounding. Start by walking short distances and then build this up.

9) Shoulder Rotations and Neck Rolls

Simply loosening your neck and shoulders can do wonders in releasing pent-up tension that prevents restful sleep. Do this in the morning when you wake up and at night before you settle down to sleep.

10) Improve Hydration to Soothe Your Metabolism

Drink enough fluids to keep yourself hydrated. Caffeine and alcohol can dehydrate you further. Do not have warm water with your meals. Excess water, cold water and water with meals weaken agni.

Food Recommendations and Steps

What I've put together through the food plan is what I call the eclectic Indo-Mediterranean diet. Let me explain. 'Indo' refers to food from India. The Mediterranean diet is food from anywhere around the Mediterranean Sea—be it Italy, France, Spain, Greece, Turkey, Lebanon, Egypt, Morocco and many more! India has a rich tradition of food in many states, each with its rich history going back centuries! So does the Mediterranean diet, which is also the diet that has been most studied by experts. While it is inclusive of so many places, and the food can be quite varied, the Mediterranean diet emphasize on high consumption of varied coloured fruits and vegetables, beans and lentils prepared in traditional ways, whole grains, seafood, small amounts of meat and poultry, and healthy fats. In this aspect, the Indian and the Mediterranean diets share a common thread for both prepare beans traditionally, and they are never a problem, unlike in the West, where beans are now vilified. There are also multiple ways to eat vegetables, where they can be the star of a meal rather than just an accompaniment. This makes both diets plant powered. Ingredients are combined in different ways, and recipes may be simple but taste delicious! Think about this diet as something from the best of blue zones—regions in the world where people are said to live the longest and the healthiest. Be eclectic and make your personal variations, as long as it stays within the framework of the programme. Flow with the creativity of cooking and dive deep into delicious taste!

Food Rules

If you are wondering whether a food item you eat is acceptable within the framework of the ten-sense protocol, you can quickly glance through the lists below. For the duration of the programme, try and avoid eating packaged food or food with artificial colouring.

Foods to Eat

1. See that every meal has fat, fibre and protein.
2. Balance your main meals of lunch and dinner based on the principles of Ayurveda. See that your plate is divided into four equal servings of a whole grain, a legume or light animal protein, a nourishing vegetable and a cleansing vegetable. Beyond this, ensure spices, healthy fats and salt are used while cooking. Reduce the proportions of the nourishing vegetables and grain if you are diabetic or prediabetic.
3. Try to balance all six tastes in every meal.
4. Spices are nature's potent healers. However, there is a subtle art to using them. They taste delicious, improve digestive health, reduce inflammation and support circulation.

5. Eat only when you are calm, relaxed and stress-free. Keep food warm and cooked as much as possible, especially in the winter. This keeps vata dosha calm.
6. Avoid most sweeteners, except for natural fruit, stevia, raw honey and coconut sugar.

Foods to Avoid

The foods below weaken agni and aggravate vata dosha.

1. Do not consume food with chemicals and chemical sweeteners, including Diet Coke, aspartame, sugar-free snacks, mints.
2. Avoid sugars as much as you can. This is an opportunity to do a sugar detox as well. If you absolutely cannot, restrict sugars to coconut sugar or stevia and avoid them altogether beyond lunchtime.
3. Restrict cheese, ice cream and pasteurized milk.
4. Limit coffee and alcohol. If you need coffee, have it after your breakfast and avoid it after morning. It is best to taper and eliminate caffeine so vata can calm down.
5. Avoid all refined oils. Cook in ghee, coconut oil, olive oil, sesame oil or home-made butter.
6. Avoid eating small meals throughout the day or snacking. Eat three meals and avoid eating in between.
7. Avoid oily and heavily spiced foods.
8. Eat whole foods only. Avoid all processed and canned foods.

Ten-sense Supplement Basics

Finding the right diet that supports sleep, while adding effective sleep supplements, can gently guide you back towards creating your own sacred sanctuary for deep blissful sleep! Remember to take one supplement at a time. Do not begin all of them together. Your body will neither be able to handle it, nor will you be able to listen to the feedback that it gives you. Begin with probiotics and magnesium. Add one every two days and observe your body's response.

Supplements Your Body Needs

Each person is unique. Even if most of us experience challenges with sleep, we cannot all take the same supplements. Though the protocol and supplements are researched and designed to work well for most people with sleep challenges, remember to stay aware and observe your own body for feedback. Consider your diet, lifestyle, stressors, routine and symptoms. In true Ayurveda, additional nutrients are not recommended. However, a body that has been struggling with poor sleep needs deficiencies corrected during a therapeutic phase before the body has been brought to a state of balance. You can use the ones recommended in the resources section of the book.

1. **Multivitamin**: Select one with methylated B vitamins, folate and bioavailable minerals. It should not contain folic acid or cyanocobalamin. A good multivitamin can support your body through stressors and can support and correct any deficiencies of trace minerals from a diet which may have been restrictive or from the years of damage that a lack of sleep might have created.
2. **Probiotics**: If you've had years of poor sleep, chances are that you have digestive distress. Probiotics can help you heal a leaky gut, improve gut motility, and support your liver in detoxification and rejuvenation. If you find yourself having

excess hunger, avoid taking any probiotics. Work with a health practitioner for this.

3. **Magnesium**: Through the programme, make sure that you take one capsule of magnesium at night. Magnesium glycinate is the best for sleep.
4. **Vitamin C**: Vitamin C supports sleep by helping to neutralize and detoxify excess cortisol. Avoid brands with sugars. Look for pure L-Ascorbic acid powder without fillers and gums.
5. **Omega-3 fatty acid**: Omega-3 is an essential fatty acid which is required as part of your diet. A high-quality fish or algal oil can provide you with it. Ghee is a great option as well.
6. **Vitamin D**: It is important to test yourself frequently and see that you have optimum levels of this vitamin. Aim for 50–80 ng/Ml. If you are low, supplement daily with a low dose for three months and then check again. Take vitamin D only in the morning.

I have come across people who try supplements and herbs without incorporating any changes to their diet and lifestyle, and they have failed completely. In such situations, more supplements only end up adding to the clean-up work of your liver. Remember to think of the different tools offered in the programme as different petals. You require all of them to make a flower!

A Typical Week-1 Day with the Ten-sense Protocol

This is a sample day to make it easier for you to apply all the information shared so far. Remember that this is still the first week, so the guidelines are basic. Sleep is critical. It's profoundly healing. If you already have included some of these steps in your life, that's fantastic; keep going!

1. **Wake Up**: Wake up naturally if you can. Take a moment to pause and do some deep breathing in your bed. *Avoid rushing to look at your phone or laptop.* Feel how soothing your sheets are on your skin. If you wake up next to someone you love, even spending a few minutes hugging them can change your whole day. Take that moment to be appreciative. The simple act of making your bed allows your brain to feel as if something has been achieved and so it can guide your actions in a similar manner all day long.
2. **Morning Routine**: A morning routine is profoundly impactful to your entire day and how you sleep. Taking that time to pause and be alone aligns you with yourself. If you have time in the morning, it is best to bring in some movement. Try some barefoot walking. If you are hesitant to go outside to a park, try to do this in your own home. Let go of feeling any embarrassment. Try to walk for half an hour without shoes, connecting to the earth, feeling grounded and rooted. After that, do some light shoulder rotations and neck movements to release tension. Try to do a warm sesame oil abhyanga two or three times this week before your bath. If exercising in the morning is challenging, try to target the evening time, before dinner. This is key in transforming your sleep. If everything together feels like too much, I suggest prioritizing the abhyanga. Do it at least once this week at any time of the day that is convenient for you.
3. **Breakfast**: Using the food rules, create your own breakfast. Don't wait to eat until you are starving, have a headache, feel jittery or angry. Usually, when you have poor sleep, you also have blood sugar imbalance. Avoid eating at a different time every day. Having meals at regular times is part of setting a strong circadian rhythm. Let breakfast be lighter in terms of

the ingredients and quantity, but with optimal protein from a lighter source. After breakfast, take your multivitamin, vitamin D and probiotics.
4. **Through the Morning**: Avoid distractions at work. Stay productive and focused, and observe your body after a balanced and satiating breakfast. The more you avoid distractions such as frequent social media check-ins, the more you will achieve in life and the less overactive your brain will be at night when you try to fall asleep. Restrict the time you spend on social media. Instal an app or use your phone settings to set a short window of time for using apps and your device. It makes a huge difference to sleep. If you keep checking your phone for a few minutes throughout the day, you are allowing your brain to keep spiking dopamine and it expects this reward often. It triggers vata imbalance through rapid movement of the eyes. This does not allow you to wind down at night or go into deep sleep. Every two hours, move around—even if it is just for a few minutes. This time between breakfast and lunch is also the best time to improve hydration. Sip on water often or have herbal teas.
5. **Lunch**: Start to add the ginger appetizer before your lunch and dinner. Lunch should be the biggest meal of the day. If you can, perhaps once this week, sit on the floor and eat your meal. It grounds you and allows for better digestion. Chew your food well. Do not eat in a rush, mindlessly. Even if your day is busy and you have just fifteen minutes, eat mindfully. Take time for gratitude before your meal. Try to eat in silence. Aim to follow the principle of a balanced plate, divided equally into whole grain, legume or animal protein, a nourishing vegetable and a cleansing vegetable, all ideally cooked with ghee and spices. If you prefer not to

use ghee, use sesame or coconut oil. This can be changed based on other aspects, such as reducing the starches in a prediabetic or diabetic state. Work with someone if you would like guidance.
6. **Through the Evening**: After your workday, if you did not get time for movement in the morning, try to do some barefoot walking for half an hour. This week, use this time to really assess and analyse what sounds in your life are disturbing you and do not serve you well. See if there are ways you can minimize them. Also explore which sounds in your life are pleasant and soothing. How can you bring more of these into your life? Just becoming aware of this is a mighty leap towards change.
7. **Dinner**: For most people, this is the meal that is the most relaxed, and can be created with love and care. If the morning and afternoon are busy, then take your time with this meal. Always make sure that you have your dinner two to three hours before bedtime. Remember that your bedtime should ideally not be later than 10 p.m. as every hour of sleep before midnight is equal to three hours of sleep after. Pitta time of the day is from 10.00 p.m. to 2.00 a.m. It is best to try and sleep before that. Just this one change can make a profound difference to the quality of your sleep. Stop looking at all devices. You require two hours without LED light so that you can produce melatonin to help you sleep. Even if you have heard that blue light has no impact, eye movement triggers vata imbalance, leading to nervous system dysregulation. Putting devices on airplane mode helps train your brain to feel safety. If you can finish a wholesome dinner before 6.00 p.m., it is great! Have your omega-3 supplement. Take your magnesium an hour before you plan to sleep. This should be 8.00 p.m. if you start winding down by 9.00.

8. **Bedtime Routine**: When you go into your bedroom, take time to enjoy the soothing space. If you have taken time to do this space, appreciate it fully. This is a space where you should feel truly safe. Smell the clean sheets and the lavender or orange oil. When you lie down, feel the softness of your sheets. Feel how your skin is soothed by it. Think about three things that you are grateful for. If you sleep near someone you love, take a few minutes to give them a deep hug. Spend two minutes taking deep abdominal breaths. Allow yourself to let go of the thoughts of your busy day. Check your nostrils. If the left nostril is closed and not active, lie on your right side to activate the parasympathetic state and help you switch off. Gently fall asleep.

Track Your Senses and Discover Where Vulnerabilities Lie

You may have already discovered which of the ten senses is vulnerable as you went through the chapters. If some chapter resonated with you, and you feel you require some deeper work with a particular sense beyond the ten-sense basic protocol, I suggest you reread that particular section or chapter a few times and see what strikes you.

In Week 2, I'll share some details about how to discover your vulnerable sense. I'll teach you how to bring protocols and practices to support that sense in the coming weeks, and how you may support it as you go beyond the four weeks. If you have completed Week 1 successfully and managed to make some changes to your diet, appreciate yourself as you've come such a long way! In Week 2, it's time to dive deeper.

Week 2

This week, you will build on the recommendations from Week 1 and go one step deeper with therapies. I also suggest that you explore how you felt with your diet and the therapies of the previous week. You are unique. If you are mindful about your body in terms of what feels better, you will feel motivated to do more. If something does not feel right, be curious and try to ask yourself why. Perhaps looking back at chapters that resonated with you can help to go deeper into specific areas that need help.

The Ten-step Plan

1. Set your circadian rhythm.
2. Begin brahmari pranayama.
3. Include aromatherapy.
4. Set the right temperature for your bedroom.
5. Start oil pulling and tongue cleaning.
6. Use castor packs.
7. Balance your pH.
8. Practise yoga.

9. Use Chinese balls.
10. Try humming.

1) Setting Your Circadian Rhythm to Soothe Sight

Take a warm bath before your dinner. It is even better if you have a warm sesame oil abhyanga before the bath. Eat a meal full of sleep-supportive vitamins and minerals after a warm bath. Set an EMF curfew every night. Go to bed at the same time every day to set your circadian rhythm. Wake up at the same time every day, even during the weekend. Get enough natural light on your retina during the day and reduce artificial light at night. Listen to guided meditations. Breathe deeply from your abdomen for five minutes every day.

2) Brahmari Pranayama to Soothe Sound

Close your eyes and relax your whole body. Your lips should be gently closed with your teeth slightly separated. Curl your hands into fists and raise them to your ears. Use your thumb to close the flap of each ear and seal off external sound. Inhale through your nostrils. As you exhale, breathe out very slowly, making a deep, steady humming sound. Do five to ten rounds at first and then increase it to fifteen minutes every day. Remember that the ears are associated with vata dosha and humming calms the sense of hearing.

3) Aromatherapy to Soothe Smell

Try mixing three drops of clary sage or geranium essential oil with one teaspoon of a carrier like coconut oil and give yourself a gentle neck rub or foot massage, as Dr Zielinski shared in the section on smell.

4) Setting the Right Temperature for Sleep

In a sleeping space, the usual recommendation is that the temperature should be between 16–21 degrees Celsius. However, this depends on body constitution, season, location, age and menstrual phase. My suggestion is to begin with abhyanga to regulate body temperature. If you are living somewhere which does not have extreme temperatures, it is best to allow the body to acclimatize naturally.

5) Oil Pulling and Tongue Cleaning

Here are the four simple steps for oil pulling:

- Measure a capful of sesame or coconut oil and add your favourite essential oil to it. I add some turmeric powder as well.
- Swish it around in your mouth for five minutes. Avoid swallowing any of it.
- Avoid spitting the oil into the sink or toilet as this can lead to clogging.
- Rinse your mouth well using water before eating or drinking anything. Brush your teeth.

For tongue cleaning, look for a stainless steel or wooden cleaner. Place it towards the back of your tongue and move it forward while applying very gentle pressure. It should bring out all the debris and bacteria. Spit out any remaining saliva and wash your mouth with warm water. Repeat this a few times.

6) Castor Packs for Detoxification

Castor oil packs can improve glutathione production. Glutathione plays a key role in liver health and detoxification. Apply a palmful of castor oil over your liver area. Your liver is under your right ribcage. Wrap an old cloth around your midriff and tie it with a soft cotton tie. Wear an old shirt and leave it on all night, or let it remain for an hour or two and then wash it off. If you menstruate, avoid this practise when you are on your period. If you live in a colder place, or if it is winter, tie a small hot water bag on top of it. Ensure that you close the cap tightly for safety. In this situation, keep it on only for 30 minutes.

7) pH Balancing to Support Uro Reproduction

Adding a few drops of lemon to your meal doesn't just help your digestion. It balances the six tastes when combined with spices. It changes the pH of your urine, preventing infections and irritable bladder.

8) Yoga for Lymphatic Movement

Suryanamaskar is a great way to stimulate lymphatic decongestion, if done correctly. Allow yourself to breathe slowly and deeply, coordinating each transitionary movement with the required breath. Remember that it is not how many you do that matters, but how you do them. Do them slowly and mindfully.

9) Chinese Balls for Stress

Hold two of them in your hands and keep rotating them, trying to change their position while they still touch each other.

Keep moving them around in different ways. More than this, I suggest including abhyanga as often as possible for it changes vata behaviour.

10) Humming

Get ready as you would for brahmari pranayama. Inhale through your nostrils, and as you exhale, breathe out very slowly, making a deep, steady, humming sound. Do five to ten rounds at first and then increase it to fifteen minutes daily.

Discover Your Vulnerable Sense

This short quiz will take you through the ten senses again and help you identify your vulnerable sense(s). Now that you have completed one week within the ten-sense protocol, it could be insightful to see if something has changed already.

Tick all the options that apply to you. The sense which receives the maximum tick marks is your most vulnerable sense. In decreasing order, you can recognize other vulnerable or slightly vulnerable senses as well. Do not consider any quiz to be foolproof. We are complex beings and cannot be boxed in by a single test or questionnaire.

Sight

1. I sleep at a different time every night.
2. I go to bed later than 10 p.m.
3. I wear sunglasses through the day.
4. I constantly check my phone and social media.
5. I watch television until I fall asleep.

6. I expose my eyes to LED light for more than an hour at a time daily.
7. I sleep at different times during the week and at the weekends.

Sound

1. I consume plenty of caffeine and alcohol.
2. I make sure I get a highly intense workout many days of the week.
3. I wake up tired and needing coffee.
4. I constantly multitask and split my focus.
5. I often skip meals.
6. I often feel anxious and fearful.
7. I eat a diet high in carbohydrates.

Smell

1. I often struggle with a stuffy nose.
2. My head often feels heavy.
3. I feel depressed and low in mood.
4. I struggle to let go of past memories.
5. I do not consume foods or supplements with omega-3.
6. I do not eat a variety of colourful plant foods.
7. I never or rarely exercise.

Touch

1. I suffer from skin-inflammatory conditions.
2. I have faced aggression or abuse.
3. I get angry easily.
4. I struggle to fall asleep when I feel hot.

5. I often wake up sweating.
6. I cannot remember when I last enjoyed hugging someone.
7. I feel repulsed at the thought of being hugged.

Taste

1. I have a bad taste in my mouth.
2. I often get teeth and gum problems.
3. I crave specific tastes.
4. I eat very fast.
5. I rarely chew my food.
6. I have never fasted or I struggle with it.
7. I drink smoothies most of the time.

Detoxification

1. I often suffer from acidity.
2. I struggle with bloating and indigestion.
3. I have many food allergies and inflammatory pains.
4. I have chronic constipation.
5. I have a bitter taste in my mouth.
6. I struggle to eat fatty foods.
7. I have hormonal challenges.

Uro Reproduction

1. I need to urinate often through the night.
2. I need to drink water through the night to avoid feeling urinary irritation.
3. I do not have a satisfying sex life.
4. I suffer from PMS.
5. I have cycle-related migraines and insomnia.

6. I experience anxiety and mood fluctuations related to my cycle.
7. I have varying symptoms through the month.

Locomotion

1. I have a belly which always looks bloated.
2. I constantly have skin allergies.
3. I suffer from a heavy head and depression.
4. I struggle with water retention.
5. I struggle to lose weight.
6. I have swelling in different parts of my body.
7. I have very little movement as part of my life.

Dexterity

1. My bones protrude in some places.
2. I have pain in my shoulders, neck, arms, hands and fingers.
3. I feel anxious and spacey.
4. I have profound pains in the winter.
5. I cannot lift anything heavy.
6. I do not feel like I have strength in my arms.
7. I have popping and cracking joints.

Speech

1. I find myself unable to say what is on my mind.
2. I often burst out, talking in ways that do not serve me.
3. I have a hoarse voice.
4. I have symptoms of low thyroid.
5. I often feel hot and sweaty.

6. I often feel cold, with icy hands and feet.
7. I have low iron.

Ten-sense Supplement Add-on for Vulnerable Sense

This is a guide to choosing an add-on supplement from this chapter. Each person is unique. Even if all of us face challenges with sleep, we cannot all take the same supplement. Even though sleep protocols and supplements are well-researched and designed to work for most, remember to stay aware and observe your own body for feedback. Consider your diet, lifestyle, stressors, routine and symptoms. Be mindful of these factors when you are considering a supplement:

1. Read the description for each supplement within the chapter of your vulnerable sense.
2. If you can pinpoint issues based on lab results or are under the care of a qualified health professional, that is best.
3. Be honest with yourself on what you truly feel you need. When confused, work with a practitioner. Remember that there is no ideal diet philosophy, and your body is truly precious and unique.
4. Choose one add-on from the list and check with an expert on how to use it safely.
5. Start taking it and observe your reactions.
6. Do not take too many supplements at the same time and avoid any if it is out of your scope to monitor symptoms.

A Typical Day in Week 2 with the Ten-sense Protocol

The sample day for Week 2 integrates all the wonderful work from Week 1 and builds on it. Keep in mind that this is not more work. You will simply be adding protocols and using them in combination with those of last week. Sleep is critical. It's profoundly healing. And remember, you matter!

1. **Wake Up**: Wake up naturally if you can. Take a moment to pause, do some brahmari breath work and humming in your bed. Avoid rushing to look at any devices. Feel how soothing your sheets are on your skin. If you wake up next to someone you love, spending a few minutes hugging them can change your whole day. Take a moment to be grateful.
2. **Morning Routine**: If you have time in the morning, this is the best time to bring in some movement. Walk barefoot. If you are hesitant to go outside to a park, try to do this in your own home. Try to walk for half an hour, connecting to the earth, feeling grounded and rooted. Do this every alternate day. On the other days, begin practising yoga. Do some light shoulder rotations and neck movements to release tension in your neck and shoulders. Practise five minutes of oil pulling while you prepare your bath and ready your clothes. If you have half an hour to spare, include a warm sesame oil abhyanga before the bath.
3. **Breakfast**: Take half a teaspoon of triphala powder mixed with half teaspoon ghee and half teaspoon honey. If you cannot take ghee or honey, mix triphala in a quarter cup of hot water. Choose your breakfast based on the food guide I've provided. Avoid eating at a different time every day. Let your meal have fat, fibre, protein and colour. Breakfast should be lighter in ingredients and quantity than other meals, but with optimal protein from a lighter source. After breakfast, take your multivitamin, vitamin D and probiotics.
4. **Through the Morning**: Every two hours, move around, rotate your shoulders and neck, or squeeze some Chinese stress balls in your hands, even if it is just for a few minutes.

The time between breakfast and lunch is also the best time to improve hydration. Sip water often or have herbal teas. Including warm hydration can be very helpful in calming vata dosha.

5. **Lunch**: Continue to eat the ginger appetizer before your lunch and dinner. Once this week, sit on the floor and eat your meal. Chew your food well. Remember that chewing eases the load on digestion. Do not eat in a rush, mindlessly. Take time for gratitude before your meal. If you feel hungry before lunch, it is a sign that your breakfast was optimal in protein and fibre. Aim to follow the principle of a balanced plate. Work with someone if you would like guidance on how to plan your meals.

6. **Through the Evening**: After your workday, if you did not get time for movement in the morning, try to do some barefoot walking or yoga for an hour. Alternate between the two. Do some brahmari breath work and humming.

7. **Dinner**: Have the ginger appetizer before your dinner. Choose your dinner with love and care. Eat dinner at a fixed time every day, two to three hours before bedtime. Remember that you should ideally go to sleep not later than 9–10 p.m. Just this one change can make a profound difference to the quality of your sleep. Putting devices on airplane mode helps train your brain to feel safety. If you can finish a wholesome dinner before 6.00 p.m., it is great! Have an omega-3 supplement. Take magnesium an hour before you plan to sleep.

8. **Night-time Routine**: Use a castor pack on your liver with a hot water bag for half an hour on as many nights as you can. When you go into your bedroom, take time to enjoy the soothing space. Bring in your favourite aromatherapy scents

into the room. When you lie down, feel the softness of your sheets. Feel how your skin is soothed by it. Think about three things that you are grateful for.

9. **Bedtime Routine**: If you sleep near someone you love, take a few minutes to hug them tight. Spend two minutes taking deep abdominal breaths. Allow yourself to let go of the thoughts of your busy day. Gently fall asleep.

Week 3

Week 3 is going to be even better because you may have started noticing changes in your sleep already, which then inspires you to go even further. This week, the therapies are a little different. If you feel better and would like to stay with what is working for you, feel free to do so.

The Ten-step Plan

1. Practice trataka.
2. Listen to a guided meditation.
3. Start jal neti.
4. Rediscover the wonderful feeling of hugging.
5. Support your vagus nerve.
6. Improve your detoxification and elimination capabilities.
7. Try squatting.
8. Practice inversions.
9. Go swimming.
10. Start journalling.

1) Practice Trataka to Strengthen Sight

Staring at a flame without blinking until your eyes tear profusely allows for glymphatic circulation. When you cannot keep your eyes open any longer, close them and let your mind be still by focusing on the image within your closed eyes. Repeat the whole process. Try this practice for fifteen minutes daily.

2) Play Guided Meditations

Choose any of the guided meditations on *The Sleep Whisperer Podcast*. It includes meditations by a few guests as well. Aim to do this once in the afternoon and once before you sleep. In the afternoon, lie down on the ground, and use earphones and an eye mask. This allows you to restrain the senses and calm down. Play a guided meditation and take a moment to pause in the middle of your day.

3) Jal Neti to Awaken Smell

You can use a copper or stainless steel neti pot. Make sure the water you use is lukewarm and as salty as your tears. Tilt your head to one side and gently pour the water through one nostril so it comes out of the other. Making a sound helps to close off the throat. Repeat it on the other side. Once you have done it on both sides, hang your head for a few moments and gently blow out the excess water through each nostril until you feel they are clear. Follow with nasyam, as described in the section on smell.

4) Hugging to Increase Oxytocin

Hugging increases oxytocin and lowers cortisol. Hugging someone you love for a few minutes can make a huge difference in your nervous system functioning.

5) Supporting Your Vagus Nerve

Switch your hot shower to a cold for a few moments at the end. It will improve your salivary production and support your sense of taste. Do not overdo this. It is best to focus on abhyanga to improve sleep.

6) Improving Detoxification and Elimination

Take half a teaspoon of triphala powder in hot water at breakfast. The bitter herbs will improve detoxification and elimination.

7) Squatting

Spend a few minutes as part of your yoga session in a squatting pose. Holding a butterfly pose will also do wonders. Take your time with hip-opening poses and acknowledge the tension within the pelvis to let go.

8) Practicing Inversions

One of the powerful ways of moving up in your yoga practice is by adding headstands and shoulder stands. You can only do these if you do not have high blood pressure. It's important to work with an experienced teacher for inversions as its common for people to injure their neck badly while trying them. A shoulder stand is gentler and passive, yet powerful in moving lymph. However, this also needs to be avoided if you have high blood pressure or neck problems like spondylitis.

9) Swimming

Swimming is simply magical. The feeling of flow and freedom that comes from feeling like a fish in water is unparalleled!

10) Journalling

Journalling whatever comes in your mind the moment you wake up allows you to maintain clarity and great awareness through the day. Writing with your non-dominant hand releases emotional suppression.

Going Deeper with Your Vulnerable Sense

Congratulations on making it to Week 3! You've come such a long way and I'm incredibly proud! I've built in wonderful protocols into the four-week plan of the ten-sense protocol, but this week, I want you to go back to the section on your vulnerable sense and look through the therapies at the last chapter there. I want you to see the whole scope of available resources to support you on an individual level.

Typical Day in Week 3

Here is a sample day for week 3, which integrates all that we have learned so far. And remember, you matter!

1. **Wake Up**: Wake up naturally if you can. Take a moment to pause and do some brahmari breath work and humming in your bed. Don't rush to look at devices. If you wake up next to someone you love, spend a few minutes hugging them. Write a one-page journal entry on anything that comes to your mind without thinking about it. This early morning brain dump releases a lot of stress that could've impeded the day.
2. **Morning Routine**: A morning routine is profoundly impactful on your entire day and how you sleep. If you have time in the morning, this is the best time to engage in some movement. Walk barefoot for at least half an hour. Alternate between a walk, yoga and swimming all through this week. When you practise yoga, include some inversions like headstand and shoulder stand if you have no contraindications. Do five minutes of oil pulling while you prepare your bath and ready your clothes. If you have the time, include a warm sesame oil abhyanga before a ten-minute soak. Soak in your bath for ten or fifteen minutes. If you do not have a bathtub, have a warm shower instead. End your shower with a one-minute cold water spray.
3. **Breakfast**: Take half a teaspoon of triphala powder and mix it with half a teaspoon each of ghee and honey. If you cannot consume ghee or honey, mix triphala in a quarter cup of hot water. Avoid eating at a different time every day. After breakfast, take your multivitamin, vitamin D and probiotics.
4. **Through the Morning**: The more you avoid distractions such as frequent social media check-ins, the more you will achieve in life. Every two hours in the day, move around and rotate your shoulders and neck. The time between breakfast and lunch is also the best time to improve hydration.

5. **Lunch**: Have the ginger appetizer before lunch. Sit on the floor whenever you can to eat your meal. Chew your food well. Take time for gratitude before your begin eating. Aim to follow the principle of a balanced plate. Have a clean, organic plant-protein shake. I have some recommendations for protein powder in the resources section.
6. **Afternoon meditation**: Try to make time for an afternoon grounding meditation of ten to fifteen minutes. Lie on the floor with an eye mask and earphones.
7. **Through the Evening**: After your workday, if you did not get time for movement in the morning, try to do some barefoot walking or yoga for an hour. Alternate between the two. Do some brahmari breath work and humming.
8. **Dinner**: Have the ginger appetizer before dinner. Choose your dinner with love and care. Remember that your bedtime should ideally not be later than 10 p.m. Aim to finish dinner by 6 p.m. Putting devices on airplane mode helps train your brain to feel safe. Take your omega-3 supplement. Have the magnesium supplement an hour before you plan to sleep.
9. **Night-time Routine**: Continue using a castor pack on your liver with a hot water bag for half an hour on as many nights as you can. Let some soothing music play for a few minutes, preferably on a timer that turns off before you start to fall asleep. Bring in your favourite aromatherapy scents into the room. Set the right temperature for your bedroom. When you lie down, feel the softness of your sheets. Think about three things that you are grateful for.
10. **Bedtime Routine**: If you sleep near someone you love, take a few minutes for a deep hug. Spend two minutes taking deep abdominal breaths. Allow yourself to let go of thoughts of your busy day. Gently fall asleep.

Week 4

By Week 4, you should have already seen tremendous changes to your sleep and to your whole life by following the ten-sense protocol. Now, it is time to envision something great for yourself, for you can now work on manifesting it with the support of great sleep! It may be interesting to go back to the quiz you did in Week 2 and see if anything has changed. Is your perspective different? Do you have a more positive outlook? Have you found yourself letting go of old memories, habits and mindsets that do not serve you well?

You can use the template for the fourth week to create your unique sleep blueprint. Build your own protocol from all that worked for you and be empowered with the knowledge that you can now restore your sleep anytime you want to.

The Ten-step Plan

1. Create your night-time routine.
2. Let go of all the disturbing sounds in your life.
3. Release old memories that do not serve you well.
4. Be with your pet.

5. Practise fasting.
6. Give yourself an enema.
7. Use a sitz bath.
8. Get a variety of movement.
9. Find your immune friends.
10. Build your breath-work blueprint.

1) Creating Your Night-time Routine

Through the last three weeks, you've gone step by step towards building a night-time routine. If you prefer doing abhyanga in the evening, prioritize half an hour for it on as many days as possible. Eat a meal full of sleep-supportive vitamins and minerals after a warm bath. Set a two- to three-hour window before bedtime with no exposure to blue light. Listen to guided meditations. Breathe deeply from your abdomen for five minutes. Never do so much that you feel overwhelmed. If you can only do one or two of these, I suggest choosing abhyanga and switching off devices before bedtime.

2) Letting Go of Disturbing Sounds

Begin by removing the sounds of electronic gadgets, whether it is television shows that are exciting and stimulating or notifications on your phone.

3) Releasing Old Memories that Do Not Serve You Well

Visualize your memories that do not serve you being tied up into a package and being sent away to the end of the world. Use guided visualizations and meditations to help you release trauma.

4) Being with Your Pet

Spending time stroking and cuddling your pet can boost oxytocin and lower cortisol.

5) Fasting

Start with twelve hours. After a few weeks, provided you are comfortable, you can increase it half an hour at a time, until you find your limit. If you have resonated with symptoms of vata imbalance, it is better that you avoid long fasts. Instead eat dinner by sunset to derive profound benefits.

6) Enema

You can buy a home enema kit, fill it with warm water and a little salt. Insert the tip into your rectum and hold the canister at a higher level for water to flow easily. Eventually, when the whole can of water enters your colon, remove the end from your body and sit on the toilet. Enemas should not become a habit. This is a one-time suggestion. If this feels out of your scope, look for colon hydrotherapy clinics or consult a skilled practitioner who can walk you through the process. Do not attempt if this does not sound comfortable to you.

7) Sitz Bath

Sitz baths bring blood circulation to the pelvis, relax internal muscles and allow more movement in the area. You require a tub which can hold water and allow you to sit so that the water comes till your waist. Fill the basin with warm water. Boil some tea. Add it to the water. When you finish, lie down for a while and bring your awareness to the sensation of blood flowing through the pelvis, and feel yourself releasing and letting go.

8) Getting a Variety of Movement

With whatever activity you do for movement, you can add variety and spice it up. Nothing feels as fresh as the simplest of changes within your movement.

9) Finding Your Immune Friends

Immune friends can be valuable resources on your journey of lowering chronic inflammation. Eat an anti-inflammatory diet, strengthen your gut, reduce alcohol, eliminate sugar and practise meditation.

10) Building Your Breathwork Blueprint

Your breath can be divided into three parts: Your inhale, your retained breath and your exhale. Fold the first two fingers of your right hand and use your thumb to close the right nostril and the ring finger to close your left nostril. When you first begin, breathe in through your left nostril counting to four, hold your breath for eight counts and then exhale through your right nostril for another eight. Repeat this with the other nostril. This is one round. Practice doing 9–15 rounds.

Another simple yet powerful practice is to breathe in through your nose, counting to four. Hold the breath gently without closing your nostrils, counting to eight. Then slowly breathe out through your mouth for another eight counts. You can also include brahmari. Find your practice by curating a breathing practice for fifteen minutes daily, decide what you want to do, the sequence and the number of rounds of each. There are guided breath sessions on *The Sleep Whisperer Podcast*, and you can follow them.

A Typical Day in Week 4

In Week 4, you will be adding to the protocols from the previous weeks and also envisioning your future goals beyond this week.

1. **Wake Up**: Wake up naturally if you can. When you open your eyes, look at the beautiful sleep space that you have created. Feel soothed by the space. Take a moment to pause, do some brahmari breath work and humming in your bed. Avoid immediately checking your devices. Write a one-page journal on anything that comes into your mind.
2. **Morning Routine**: Continue alternating between a walk, yoga and swimming if you have time to move in the morning. Spending time with your pet is another great way to get some exercise. Include inversions like headstand and shoulder stand to your yoga routine if you have no contraindications. Do five minutes of oil pulling while you prepare your bath and ready your clothes. Let your favourite soothing music play in the room while you get ready. Do jal neti before you shower. If you have time, do a warm sesame oil abhyanga before your bath. Do an enema just once this week. The day you do the enema, have a warm shower. Do this just once and not every week.
3. **Breakfast**: Continue taking triphala in the morning. You are setting a strong circadian rhythm and having meals at regular

times is part of this. Incorporate some fasting to your day. Try to maintain a fourteen-hour gap between dinner and breakfast. This will happen naturally if you finish dinner close to sunset. Try to have fat, fibre, protein and colour at every meal. After breakfast, take your multivitamin, vitamin D and probiotics.

4. **Through the Morning**: Every two hours, move around, rotate your shoulders and neck, or squeeze some Chinese stress balls, even if it is just for a few minutes. Sip water often or have herbal teas.

5. **Lunch**: Have the ginger appetizer before lunch. If you can, perhaps once this week, sit on the floor and eat your meal. Chew your food well. Start your mealtime with gratitude. Aim for a balanced plate and continue having a clean, organic plant-protein shake. Practice an afternoon grounding meditation for ten to fifteen minutes.

6. **Through the Evening**: After your workday, if you did not get time for movement in the morning, try to do some barefoot walking or yoga for an hour. Alternate between the two. Do some brahmari breath work and humming. Ten minutes of breathing practice can be followed by a short meditation. Towards the end of your meditation, become aware of the old memories that do not serve you and release them.

7. **Dinner**: Have the ginger appetizer before dinner. Choose your dinner with love and care. Finish eating before 6 p.m. Remember that your bedtime should ideally not be later than 10 p.m. Switch off from devices and focus on calming practices such as breathing, guided meditations or spending time with your loved ones.

8. **Night-time Routine**: When you go into your bedroom, take time to enjoy the soothing space. Let some relaxing music play for a few minutes. Use your favourite aromatherapy

scents into the room. When you lie down, feel the softness of your sheets. Think about three things that you are grateful for.
9. **Bedtime Routine**: If you sleep near someone you love, take a few minutes to embrace them. Spend two minutes taking deep abdominal breaths. Allow yourself to let go of the thoughts of your busy day. Gently fall asleep.

Going Forward with the Ten-sense Protocol

You've come such a long way! Examine where you started and how you felt then by looking back at what you wrote at the start. Write down how you feel now and all that has changed within you. Acknowledge the work that you have done and offer gratitude for everything that supported you through the transformation process.

You can continue following the protocol for the fourth week or build your own routine based on what you feel requires the most support and what felt healing for you in the last four weeks. Congratulations on your great work!

Supporting Your Vulnerable Sense: A Quick Glance Guide

Sight

1. Expose your retina to daylight during the day.
2. Wear blue-light blockers after sunset.
3. Practice trataka.
4. Restrict social media usage.
5. Avoid having a television in your bedroom.
6. Sleep at the same time through the week.
7. Do some eye exercises.

Sound

1. Avoid overtraining and heavy exercise.
2. Reduce loud sounds in the evening.
3. Do not skip meals or fast.
4. Eat a diet that is as diverse and restriction-free as possible.
5. Eat more proteins and fats.
6. Practice brahmari or humming.
7. Listen to the sound of silence.

Smell

1. Eat more colour in your food.
2. Increase omega-3 foods. Add fish to your diet if necessary. If you are vegetarian, ghee is adequate. If you are vegan, include some seaweed.
3. Move your body.
4. Release old memories.
5. Spend time with those who make you laugh.
6. Learn sutra neti and jal neti.
7. Breathe deeply.

Touch

1. Have a cold bath or go for a swim.
2. Massage your whole body with castor oil.
3. Spend time hugging someone you love.
4. Stroke your pet.
5. Apply aloe vera on your body.
6. Find foods that work for you, not those your friend suggests.
7. Practise yoga.

Taste

1. Have zinc supplements.
2. Be consistent with oil pulling. Add some drops of tea tree oil.
3. Eat slowly and mindfully.
4. Try a day of fasting.
5. Have a cold shower.
6. Consume neem.
7. Include all flavours in meals.

Detoxification

1. Avoid fruit with your meals.
2. Add spices to your meals.
3. Rub castor oil on your body before a bath.
4. Do an enema with salt water, but no more than once.
5. Have fixed mealtimes. You should have your last meal by sunset.
6. Eat more plant foods.
7. Eat beets.

Uro Reproduction

1. Eat foods that are more alkaline, such as fruits and vegetables.
2. Have warm beverages between meals.
3. Avoid alcohol and caffeine.
4. Do a sitz bath.
5. Have balanced meals that support healthy hormones.
6. Increase omega-3 consumption.
7. Soak in cold water.

Locomotion

1. Engage in one form of movement every day.
2. Avoid heavy exercise.
3. Practice swimming, walking and yoga.
4. Commit to a daily practice of sun salutations.
5. Go for a dance class.
6. Walk barefoot.
7. Stand upside down.

Dexterity

1. Do shoulder and neck exercises.
2. Increase omega-3 intake.
3. Wean yourself off painkillers.
4. Include standing exercises that move your arms.
5. Go for a walk, swinging the arms.
6. Do exercises like planks to build arm strength.
7. Try knitting and sewing.

Speech

1. Gargle with salt and turmeric water.
2. Journal every single day.
3. Find someone with whom you can share every emotion.
4. Eat iron-rich foods.
5. Soak in cold water.
6. Eat a variety of vegetables.
7. Ensure you consume enough protein.

39

How to Choose a Sleeping Position

I cannot conclude this book without a chapter on sleeping positions. There is so much advice readily available on ideal sleeping positions. However, I think that there is a lot more to this. The ideal sleeping position is based on each person's body, their level of stress and much more.

1. Sleeping on your back is possibly the healthiest as it maintains a neutral position for the spine. It is not ideal if you have sleep apnoea or difficulty breathing as it can close the airway and increase snoring. It's not the most popular position. I divide this position into several variations. The *shavasana version* allows your forearm muscles to be in an open position that is more conducive to relaxation. The *baby position* has your arms over your head and can promote a feeling of being free. *Palms on the abdomen* can help breath work and ease the shift from a sympathetic nervous system. The *tree version* is sleeping with one leg folded. It can affect those with sciatica. But if you feel relaxed, you can keep a pillow under the knee to not stress the hip. If you sleep with both legs folded and arms over your head like a baby, it can feel relaxing on the back.

Anything on your back can be easy to physically let go. But this requires you to feel some form of safety and trust. Lying with your body facing the world is innately vulnerable and, if you have insecurity, it can make it difficult for you to feel safe in this position. Sleeping on the back is calming to vata dosha. Make sure to cover your head and ears.

2. Lying on your side is easier on your neck and back. It is also easier if you are prone to snoring. In our ancient traditions, this was known as matsyakridasana, or flapping fish. Your bottom leg is straight with your top leg folded over. You can then rest your neck and head on a soft pillow. It eases your legs, perineum and lower back, and promotes sleep. Overall, it is restorative for the entire body. It relaxes a lot of tension in the sacral, lumbar and hips. It can be a great sleeping position for many people, including those struggling with back pain. It is absolutely the best one for pregnancy. It relieves sciatic pain by relaxing the muscles of the legs.

3. Surprisingly, the foetal position is the most popular sleeping position. However, it can restrict breathing in your diaphragm and leave you feeling a bit sore in the morning if you are prone to pain. You can reduce strain on your hips by placing a pillow between your knees. If you have eaten too close to bedtime, or if you have eaten a very heavy meal, then this is not really the position to use. It can compress the abdomen and put a lot of stress on digestion, leading to heartburn if you are prone to it.

4. Lying on the abdomen can feel safe for many. While this is good for easing snoring, it's bad for your neck. You may wake up feeling stiff. Ancient wisdom and yoga say something different about this. Lying on your abdomen with hands folded in front and resting your cheek can be deeply

relaxing. The breath creates a gentle rocking movement at the abdomen, which allows you to soothe and gently massage the abdominal area. It allows you to fall into the earth. It is a great sleeping position if you struggle with ovulatory or menstrual cramps. Try joining the tips of your forefinger and the tips of your thumb together to form a spade. Place your hands under your hip with your palms facing the body. This allows your hip to rest in the cradle of your palms and soothes cramping. Usually, lying on the abdomen is also helpful if someone feels vulnerable to lie down facing the sky.

5. Understanding the science of the breath is important as well. Your right nostril represents the sympathetic nervous system. The left nostril represents the parasympathetic nervous system. Sleeping on the left with your right nostril facing up promotes lymph drainage from the brain, and is especially useful if you are prone to lymphatic congestion and even depression. It is easier on you heart and helps bile flow better. It is also a great position if you are going to bed with a full stomach. It calms kapha dosha. If you have an active mind, then you may have an easier time falling asleep by turning to the right side. If you have a full stomach, then you should lie down with your right nostril up. If your mind is too alert and sympathetic, lie down with the left nostril up to activate the parasympathetic system. This is calming to pitta dosha. Weather can influence this flow. Cold weather triggers a parasympathetic response and you turn to the left, which is probably why you sleep a lot more in winter. Hot activates the sympathetic and prevents sleep. Meditation can balance both.

6. If you struggle with back issues, then lying on your side may be better. If you struggle with reflux or a similar condition, you can't lie on the abdomen. If you are pregnant, then you

can't lie on your back or on your abdomen. Do you have pain in the neck? Do you struggle with a stuffy sinus? Then lying on the back can make it worse and impact breathing. If you struggle with high levels of stress, you may want to adopt a position that is parasympathetic. What about whether you share a bed? Is the other person someone who hugs? That can change the position altogether. A lot of research has shown that couples who truly feel connected hug each other for a while and sleep in positions that's most comfortable for them individually.

It is great to practise abdominal breathing on your back to balance the two hemispheres. It exerts a calming influence on cardiac function and improves oxygenation of blood, which triggers a shift to a parasympathetic system, away from fight or flight. Once you do this for ten minutes, you can shift to a more comfortable position. The main thing to consider is a full stomach versus an active mind while choosing a side to lie on. If you have physical challenges, take your time finding what's most comfortable for you. Ultimately, you can also allow your instinct and comfort to guide your choice. Keep in mind that during sleep you will slip into any position and that is perfectly fine!

40

Eating for Good Sleep

The concept of the balanced plate from Ayurveda will be helpful for most people unless there are specific challenges or allergies which require customization. These can include being diabetic, prediabetic, having insulin resistance, being unable to tolerate grains, etc. There are several recipes for colourful plant foods rich in phytonutrients. I've chosen the cleanest proteins like grass-fed lamb, wild-caught fish and legumes in the recipes I have provided on my website. I have also included some notes with each recipe, so do make sure to read them to avoid any food reactions. Remember that each body is truly unique. Try to remove alcohol and caffeine when following the four-week plan or keep them to a minimum. I've also included tons of anti-inflammatory spices. If you do not like the recipes, please feel free to create your own. Just make sure to follow the food recommendations in the ten-sense protocol. You can get all my recipes as a downloadable e-book on my website at https://ohahealth.com/sleep-book-bonus

Remember, my food mantra is fat, fibre, protein and colour! If you can tolerate grains, they can be easily included in the framework of a balanced bowl.

General Meal Guidelines

1. Eat a grounding and warm breakfast with a light plant-protein shake, if you require it.
2. Having warm, cooked sweet potato with ghee, spices and baby spinach, along with a plant protein shake, will give you adequate protein at breakfast, while keeping the meal balanced.
3. We are all unique and our agni may be different at different times. However, it is best to have lunch around noon as the heaviest meal of the day.
4. Nourishing your body with the right balance prevents illness and promotes vibrant health. Augmenting foods are nourishing and grounding. They add to the body and enhance vitality. The primary taste of augmenting food is madhura, or sweet. Sour and salt are also slightly augmenting. Extractive foods are cleansing in nature and require the body to give up something to digest them. Digesting extractive foods breaks down the essential fats for healthy functioning of body and mind. The result is a lighter feeling in the body. Extractive tastes are pungent, bitter and astringent. Use healthy fats and simmer salt and spices in the fat before adding other ingredients. The final plate should have equal portions of a cooked whole grain, cooked legume or animal protein, nourishing vegetable and cleansing vegetable respectively.
5. In an Indian meal, this framework can be as simple as a plate which has a quarter each of brown rice, rajma, palak and sweet potatoes or a plate with barley, mung dal, cauliflower and carrot; millet, fish curry, cabbage and lauki; or khichdi with mung dal, brown rice, sweet potatoes and spinach.

6. Please change the proportion based on individual requirements such as being prediabetic or diabetic. If you have such restrictions, please reach out for consultation with me.
7. Soups are best combined with whole grains or grounding foods to avoid weakening agni. Just like smoothies, a meal which is a watery soup can result in the excess water putting out the fire in you.
8. Have fixed mealtimes. Finish dinner by sunset. Have ingredients that are relatively easy to digest for your last meal. You might have heard of eating a small amount of protein (such as a piece of chicken/pumpkin seeds/nut butter last thing at night before sleeping. This is called a protein 'pill'. However, if your overall food is balanced, you need not do so.

The Ten-sense Plate Framework

I want you to respect your tastes, tradition and culture while following the practices here, for these play a major role in creating food memories that serve you. These frameworks can help you can create your own plate.

1. Follow the meal mantra of fat, fibre, protein and colour with every meal. Aim for each meal to have two vegetables, a source of protein, healthy fats and fibre. Follow the balanced plate guidelines and create your own.
2. Let your fat intake be from ghee, nuts, olive oil, coconut oil, coconut milk, avocado and nut milks. Proteins can include lamb, bone broth, collagen, fish, lentils, beans, nuts and seeds. For carbohydrates, turn to millets, quinoa, amaranth, buckwheat, ragi, brown rice, black rice, sweet potatoes,

yellow pumpkins and cauliflower. Follow the balanced bowl framework if you are not diabetic, prediabetic or insulin resistant.

3. Digestion is the source of so many ailments, including inflammation. Chewing supports digestion tremendously, and oil pulling regulates your tastebuds and mouth microbiome. Follow recommendations for healthy agni.
4. It is best to have a warm breakfast. Eat only until the first burp. The magical sleep plate begins at breakfast. Lunch should be the main meal. Combine it with a clean plant-protein shake.
5. When it comes to fluids, see that you have plenty that are not processed, sugary or stimulating. Drink herbal teas and warm water.
6. If you have issues with blood sugar and insulin, which can be a reason for belly fat, getting angry if you miss meals, frequent headaches and sleep troubles, lower your intake of grains and sugary carbohydrates for some time. Let your meals be more vegetables, some whole grains, protein and fat.
7. Think of following a more pescatarian diet if you are a non-vegetarian. I prefer that you avoid poultry as it is not a great source of protein, especially in India.
8. Soy is a phytoestrogen, which is not ideal. Small amounts of miso, tempeh, tamari and organic non-GMO tofu are acceptable.
9. Consume cooked vegetables through soups, stir-fry and stews, rather than salads and smoothies.
10. Avoid raw salads. If you do enjoy one occasionally, follow the guidelines for a balanced plate and eat it warm or at room temperature, with cooked vegetables.
11. If you can tolerate organic whole wheat, have it at lunch when agni is strong.

12. Kebabs are great since they have protein, vegetables and spices. Make sure that your animal protein is grass-fed. Avoid poultry and stay with grass-fed red meat or wild caught and freshwater fish. Combining them with a salad or soup will complete a meal.
13. Herb butter, seed spread, hummus and avocado are great fats to regulate blood sugar. You can use ghee or coconut oil to sauté your vegetables or protein. Chutneys and dips like hummus are nutrient-rich ways to balance any meal. Spreads and dips like hummus or cashew coriander can be combined with protein and vegetables to complete the meal. It can also be used as a spread on a whole-wheat or gluten-free sandwich or roti and topped with vegetables to complete a meal. Once you understand that you need to bring in adequate fat, fibre, protein and colour to every meal, you are a food star!

Resources

Here is a list of my recommendations for supplements. Please consult a skilled practitioner to implement them safely.

1. **Multivitamin:** Pure Encapsulations, Designs for Health, Life Extension or any reputable brand without folic acid and cyanocobalamin
2. **Probiotics**: Microbiome Labs MegaSporeBiotic or Zenbiome, Econorm
3. **Magnesium**: Magnesium Glycinate from Pure Encapsulations, Trexgenics or any reputable brand
4. **Vitamin C**: L-Ascorbic acid from Sharrets or any reputable brand
5. **Omega-3 Essential Fatty Acid**: Ancient Nutrition, Nordic Naturals, Pure Encapsulations, Kirkland or any reputable brand
6. **Vitamin D**: Any brand from a reputable source
7. **Other nutrients**: Please look for reputable brands globally, as suggested above, or consult a practitioner.
8. **Circadian Therapy Glasses**: https://vivarays.com?sca_ref=1132978.lTmZvKjZ2k

9. **Essential oils**: dōTERRA, Kama Ayurveda, RAS, Vibrant Blue Oils or any reputable brand
10. **DNA testing for functional impact of sleep**: DNA360 by the DNA Company. Use thednacompany.com/ancientsleep to avail a $80 discount.
11. **Plant-protein powder**: Sunwarrior, Truvani, Ancient Nutrition, Origin Nutrition or any brand that is free of soy, dairy, gluten and sugar

Acknowledgements

Writing a book was way harder than I thought and it is with immense gratitude that I conclude this one. I place this book as an offering at the feet of Krishna, the Divine Blue God. My eyes see you in Guruvayoor every moment. There is a renowned Sanskrit verse that beautifully defines what I feel.

yatkritaṁ yatkariṣhyāmi tatsarvaṁ na mayā kritamtvayā kritaṁ tu phalabhuk tvameva madhusūdana

What all the karmas that I have done, and all the ones that I will do, Madhusudana, it is only you that does them all, and enjoys their fruits.

—Veda Vyasa, translated by Gita Press

To Divine Mother Mookambika, for her protection and eternal guidance. The day we printed out this manuscript years ago and placed it at your altar for blessings, I knew there was no other path for this book.

ACKNOWLEDGEMENTS

To Swami Sivananda, Swami Vishnudevananda, Swami Govindananda, Mahavatar Babaji and Swami Virajananda—for grace.

To Mark Malatesta of Literary Agent Undercover. I never knew that the call I booked with the very last bit of my money would transform my life. Your valuable advice on the changes I needed to make so that an esteemed literary agent would trust me was beyond invaluable. The visualization you walked me through about receiving a call from one of the top global publishers feels like a miracle of manifestation when it did happen.

To Jayapriya Vasudevan. Tears well up in my eyes as I write this section. Not only did you show trust in me, but went beyond what anyone else would have. There are simply no words to express my gratitude. I hope that I have a chance to repay you. My heart is full of love for you. I don't think I could ever have been blessed with a better literary agent.

To Sonal Nerurkar, who fought to have this book acquired. Please know that you being a warrior for me will never be forgotten.

To HarperCollins India for having faith in this book. Mark Malatesta asked me one day, much later, what I did to celebrate this acquisition. My response was that I relaxed one afternoon. I think I was still in shock. The words Mark said to me made me shiver. He asked me if I knew what it was to be accepted by one of the top publishers in the world. Thank you for placing your trust in me.

To Trisha Bora, senior commissioning editor at HarperCollins India, for being the very best guide through this journey. As someone who struggles to navigate big changes and spirals into stress when I need to go out of my comfort zone, you always held my hand gently. Thank you for all that you coaxed me into changing in this book so that it would be better.

Acknowledgements

To Dhru Purohit, for everything. Your belief in me when I was nothing at all is something I hold immense gratitude for. Your trust, guidance and support are truly life's blessings. To Dr Mark Hyman, for taking the time to write the foreword to this book amidst all the brilliant things that he does. Thank you several times over.

To my mentors through this journey of healing. Andrea Nakayama, for teaching me the concept of 'it depends'. To Dr Deanna Minich, for shining a light on positive presentation and teaching me never to put anyone down to climb up. To Myra Lewin, for reminding me that health is simple and we do not need to overthink it. To all the other teachers on this journey. All of you live firmly in my heart. I would be nothing without you.

To Nanditha Krishna, for inspiring me with how strongly you hold the sacred knowledge of India, as a woman, and for taking the time to write such a beautiful foreword to this book. I am indeed grateful, aunty. To Prashanth Krishna—growing up with you was destiny. Having you as a true friend for life is a blessing.

To the authors who have contributed to this book. The warmth and support you showed to me is wonderful. Dr Michael Murray, that someone of your experience would support me is invaluable. Dr Deanna Minich, you radiate goodness and warmth. Kiran Krishnan, you amaze me with all that you do while retaining your simplicity and graciousness. Sachin Patel, beyond everything else, you are first a great human being. Dr Eric Zielinski, that you still remain humble and good is inspiring. Roudy Nassif, I love that we always support each other, and more than that, you are a dear friend.

To Rekha Saleela Nair, for walking with me in my journey of rebranding myself. Your curiosity and wonder at why I chose not to shine for what I do sparked us on a joint journey of self-discovery. To Suparna Umashankar, for your patient legal advice through my forgetful badgering. Thank you both for being part of my inner circle and the truest of friends.

To K.L. Mukesh, thank you for mentoring me and for choosing to be in my life. You are and will always be the calm voice in my head whenever I feel overwhelmed. You are truly the brother of my heart. To Purna, for being patient with me and always nurturing me with the right advice like a mother.

To my mother Prabha Kannan, thank you for sparking within me the love for reading and books and for all those years of taking me to Landmark after school. To my father, the late M.N. Kannan, thank you for teaching me the value of hard work and always understanding when I was overwhelmed. Tears rolled down your cheeks the day I told you this book had been acquired by HarperCollins India. Today, tears roll down my cheeks that you are not around. However, I know in my heart that you are watching and smiling proudly, wherever you are. To my beloved grandfather, V.K. Rangaswamy, son of V.T. Krishnamachari, for teaching us all the wisdom that lies within the magical realm of books. To my sister, Rekhs, for always being there for me with no judgement.

To my mother-in-law, Parvathy Amma, for showering me with the love shown to a daughter and for accepting me just as I was.

This book would never be a reality without my two boys. Shyam, the day I walked into that store and our eyes met was truly the day I was reborn. You entering my life, peeled away all my layers and revealed my true radiant self. Your spiritual guidance sparked the light of this book. There are so many incidents that give me goosebumps when I think of them. You are truly the one who has made me who I am today. This book is as much yours as it is mine. Omkar, I yearned for a child for decades, and then I heard a voice in my head telling me my patience will pay off because an extremely special soul was waiting to be born through me. You are truly that blessing. Your birth has truly revealed my purpose. You are beyond special.

I don't think we truly celebrate and appreciate ourselves enough. I celebrate myself. Staying steadfast with truth amidst arduously testing times has been the cornerstone of who I am. This book is a testimony that staying on the path of truth always pays off.

This book would mean nothing to me without you reading it. I thank you for choosing the book and for giving it your time. I'm so glad that our paths have crossed. Connections can be formed in any way but there is none as real as a physical meeting. If we ever connect, please share with me how my book helped you and in what way it transformed your life. Do share it with others as well. There are probably thousands, even millions, of people struggling with sleep, who lie in that gap of the sleep-care paradigm and are, therefore, struggling with their life even in this moment. By sharing the information in this book, you could save someone in many ways. After all, paying it forward can be the way that we can all change the world, one step at a time.

Notes

Scan this QR code to access the detailed notes

About the Author

Deepa Kannan is an Allied Functional Medicine practitioner, Ayurvedic health counsellor and yogini. She focuses on merging the deep science of functional medicine with the ancient wisdom of yoga and Ayurveda through her practice, OHA. Having a son with an adrenal condition gave her a deep insight into the working of the adrenals and the stress response as it relates to all health and sleep. Her articles have been shared by Dr Mark Hyman, MD, a fourteen-time *New York Times* bestselling author. She also gave the opening speech on Health Hacks at Amazon Web Services and YourStory HeathTech 2019 to the heads of healthcare start-ups in India. She has been featured on the award-winning podcast *15-Minute Matrix* and UK Health Radio.

HarperCollins *Publishers* India

At HarperCollins India, we believe in telling the best stories and finding the widest readership for our books in every format possible. We started publishing in 1992; a great deal has changed since then, but what has remained constant is the passion with which our authors write their books, the love with which readers receive them, and the sheer joy and excitement that we as publishers feel in being a part of the publishing process.

Over the years, we've had the pleasure of publishing some of the finest writing from the subcontinent and around the world, including several award-winning titles and some of the biggest bestsellers in India's publishing history. But nothing has meant more to us than the fact that millions of people have read the books we published, and that somewhere, a book of ours might have made a difference.

As we look to the future, we go back to that one word—a word which has been a driving force for us all these years.

Read.

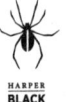